FREEDOM
from
FIBROMYALGIA

THE **5** WEEK

PROGRAM PROVEN TO CONQUER PAIN

FREEDOM

from

FIBROMYALGIA

THE **5** WEEK

PROGRAM PROVEN TO CONQUER PAIN

Nancy Selfridge, M.D.,
& Franklynn Peterson

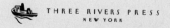

THREE RIVERS PRESS
NEW YORK

Writing this book to combine both our voices and points of view sometimes posed a problem. We have sometimes had to switch among we, I, Dr. Selfridge, Nancy, and Franklynn.

Because some people feel stigmatized by fibromyalgia, we've preserved the anonymity of those who have shared their stories by changing all names and identifying characteristics. But their feelings and experiences are authentic and presented as they were told to us. We want to thank them for their openness, honesty, and help in developing the techniques and exercises for overcoming fibromyalgia that are an essential part of this book.

Finally, this book is not intended as a substitute for a physician's care; no book can do that. We hope you'll share this book with your doctor so the two of you can be more effective partners in your health care.

Published by Three Rivers Press, New York, New York.
Member of the Crown Publishing Group.

Random House, Inc. New York, Toronto, London, Sydney, Auckland
www.randomhouse.com

THREE RIVERS PRESS is a registered trademark and the Three Rivers colophon is a trademark of Random House, Inc.

Printed in the United States of America

Design by Elina D. Nudelman

Author photograph: Jay Jurado

Library of Congress Cataloging-in-Publication Data
Selfridge, Nancy.
    Freedom from fibromyalgia: the 5-week program proven to conquer pain / Nancy Selfridge and Franklynn Peterson.—1st ed.
        Includes bibliographical references.
        1. Fibromyalgia—Psychosomatic aspects. 2. Fibromyalgia—Alternative treatment. 3. Mind and body therapies.   I. Peterson, Franklynn.   II. Title.
RC927.3 .S455 2001
616.7′4—dc21   00-046668

ISBN 0-8129-3375-3

10 9 8 7 6 5 4 3 2 1

First Edition

To my fibromyalgia patients. Your stories convinced me of the mind/body nature of our symptoms and kept me searching for a cure.

—Nancy Selfridge

To Harry Kniaz, M.D. I wish everybody could find doctors as intelligent, intuitive, and caring as Harry, and find friends who are as much fun. I feel blessed to have found both in one very special mensch.

—Franklynn Peterson

CONTENTS

Foreword   ix

PART 1: UNDERSTANDING FIBROMYALGIA   **1**

CHAPTER 1   Fibromyalgia: Misunderstood,
Misdiagnosed Misery   3

CHAPTER 2   Eight Fibromyalgia Fables   24

CHAPTER 3   Fibromyalgia 101: What It Is   40

PART 2: TOOLS TO BATTLE FIBROMYALGIA   **65**

CHAPTER 4   Put Your New Knowledge to Work   67

CHAPTER 5   Simplify: Make Room to Get Better   101

CHAPTER 6   Meditate to Access Your Mind   112

CHAPTER 7   Cut Old Angers Down to Size   126

CHAPTER 8   Journaling, Self-Talk, and
Visualization   147

CHAPTER 9   Put Your Dreams to Work   174

PART 3:   THE FIVE-WEEK PLAN TO HEAL
          FIBROMYALGIA   185

CHAPTER 10   Week One: Plan to Heal
             Fibromyalgia   187

CHAPTER 11   Week Two: Show Your Brain
             and Body Who's Boss   204

CHAPTER 12   Week Three: Teach Your Brain
             and Body to Live with Rage   208

CHAPTER 13   Week Four: Time to Start Feeling
             Really Good Again   223

CHAPTER 14   Week Five: Make Your Freedom
             from Fibromyalgia Last   238

             Notes   250
             Resources   252
             Acknowledgments   255
             Index   256

I am pleased to introduce this important book to the reading public. We are in the midst of a number of epidemics in the United States that are a direct result of the failure of the North American medical community to recognize the cause of these epidemics. It is as though the doctors had suddenly decided that the germ theory of disease was no longer valid. In this case, they have decided that a variety of pain disorders that are clearly based on the interplay of everyday human emotions with physical reactions are due either to some mysterious chemical reaction or physical concomitants, like repetitive stress in the workplace.

One of these disorders is a condition that affects millions of American women that goes by the medical name of fibromyalgia. This condition has become epidemic in the last fifteen years or so and immediately prompts the question: What has happened to explain this new epidemic? The human race has been around for hundreds of thousands of years. Why is there an epidemic of fibromyalgia now?

The answer is simple. Because it is a mind-body disorder that will spread in epidemic fashion if it is not recognized as such, and that is what has happened in the United States.

Dr. Selfridge and Mr. Peterson have suffered from this disorder and have recovered from it because they came to know the true nature of the problem. Now they want to share their knowledge of this devastating condition and what they did to get over it.

This is a very important book, for there are very few people, in or out of the medical community, who truly understand what fibromyalgia is all about. Dr. Selfridge and Mr. Peterson are pioneers—and their experience and their advice are both in the tradition of pioneers, whose mission it is to reveal the truth—and humanitarians, strongly motivated to help those who are in trouble and in need of guidance and help.

Not everyone can profit from their message, but there are millions who will. I salute them for their courage and their devotion to the needs of people who suffer the disabling consequences of pain, in this case the pain of fibromyalgia.

—John Sarno, M.D.

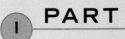

PART

I

UNDERSTANDING

FIBROMYALGIA

Jean: I don't need a doctor, doctors invent
              illnesses that don't exist.
Berenger: Perhaps they do . . . but after they
              invent them, they cure them.
                        —Eugène Ionesco

FIBROMYALGIA: 1
MISUNDERSTOOD, MISDIAGNOSED
MISERY

Come travel with us through the depths and over the peaks of one of the most mystifying sets of symptoms known to modern medicine: those of fibromyalgia. This disease is also among the most painful—whole-body pain without letup, without a pause. The authors are all too familiar with this pain, though we've been free of it for over two years. Each of us suffered with fibromyalgia over what seemed to be the longest, most tedious decades of our lives. Nancy has given birth to two delightful daughters and has had surgeries and has broken bones, yet her pain from fibromyalgia was worse. Frank has been divorced twice, but the stress and turmoil of those family wars was no match for fibromyalgia.

Fibromyalgia now rides on the backs of at least four million Americans, about 2 percent of our population. Many know what it's called; many are still undiagnosed, or diagnosed incorrectly with every malady from arthritis to tendonitis. The National Institute of Arthritis and Musculoskeletal and Skin Diseases (NIAMS) repeats figures counted by the conservative American College of Rheumatology: three million to six million cases in the United States.[1] Overall, 3.4 percent of women struggle with the illness, including about 7 percent of women between sixty and seventy-nine years old.[2] Men are not immune; maybe they're just more reticent to come forward to have their symptoms diagnosed.

Fibromyalgia knows no racial boundaries. It also knows no geographic boundaries. Two percent of the world gets up every morning unrested and sore and goes to bed very early every evening still exhausted, still sore.

After a few years with fibromyalgia, the tears may stop flowing while the pain pounds on. On some days, in self-defense, the mind spreads a confusing balm over the brain that makes it seem as if the pain is subsiding. But it also seems to slow down thinking. Though doctors don't yet have a name for this common experience, fibromyalgia sufferers call it "fibro fog." When fibro fog comes on, the senses seem powered by a nearly dead battery. Our tongues feel thick and stiff, unruly; our eyes seem veiled in gauze. Coordination lapses. We drop things. We stumble, sometimes seeming to look like drunks. Our brains don't even feel as if they're connected to themselves. Words get lost. Memory skids. Thoughts seem to slow down and seize up.

Many of us welcome this fibro fog because it seems the only respite available from our near-constant pain—quicker than the lidocaine and methadone some doctors have prescribed, more relaxing than the spinal blocks others have tried. Yet when researchers try to find out exactly what causes the fog or how it works, they've found it elusive. Neuropsychiatric testing often turns up nothing abnormal or a vague increase in distractibility.

Nobody has ever directly died of fibromyalgia. But neither has anybody really lived with it. It takes over every life it enters. It may grudgingly retreat, but not far, when attacked with the best painkillers known to modern science. A common scene at a local fibromyalgia support group is the youngish fibromyalgia sufferer dragging her shiny steel hospital-issue intravenous support. Day and night, it drips the soothing painkiller lidocaine into her veins.

Fibromyalgia can make people desperate. Probably the most controversial were the reported euthanasia patients of Dr. Jack Kevorkian, Michigan's "Dr. Death," who were fibromyalgia sufferers seeking relief from constant pain. We should at least thank Dr. Kevorkian for believing that their pain was real; so many of his peers pirouette away, not sensing that a soul could be so exhausted, it feels it can't live another night with fibromyalgia. But we wrote this book to give fibromyalgia sufferers hope so that you'll choose life. We hope its message will inspire and support those of you who feel like you've been trapped in hell for years.

Fibromyalgia does strike some youngsters. Dr. Selfridge had it in her teens. But the average age of onset is in middle age. It mostly hits people who've led full lives, compulsively working at a career, having a family, and joining the PTA, often delaying the fun things for later. But once fibromyalgia hits, there is no later. The pain traps you in the moment, and as it digs deeper, the future can become too painful to contemplate.

Family and friends of fibromyalgia victims often go through another kind of hell. They watch the pain, helpless to make it go away, even helpless to distract the sufferer long enough to enjoy a bit of life. They hear conflicting stories from doctors, read conflicting stories in the popular press; they become conflicted, sensing the pain their loved one bears while once-trusted authorities declare that the pain isn't real, that the illness is all in the head. The fibromyalgia victim is often blamed and isolated, and sometimes divorced or abandoned. Alienated by prejudices, misinformation, and conflicting opinions by half-informed family members, doctors, social workers, and insurance claim adjusters, fibromyalgia sufferers find themselves shunted onto islands of isolation with only other fibromyalgia sufferers for company—and believe us, we're not often good company.

When you add up these sufferers and include their immediate families, at least 6 percent of the world's population live greatly diminished lives because of fibromyalgia—ten million to twenty million people in the United States alone, five hundred million throughout the world. In northern England, 11.2 percent of adults suffer with chronic widespread pain like that of fibromyalgia.[3]

Fibromyalgia saps an estimated $24 billion from the U.S. economy every year in lost wages. Up to another $4 billion is wasted on unsuccessful conventional treatments; additional millions are spent on herbs, massages, acupuncture, audiotapes, and underground medications. When Franklynn heard that there was no cure for fibromyalgia, he headed for the health food and vitamin department of a large supermarket with only one question: Should he start at the A end of the shelf or at the Z end? He grabbed a bottle of arginine. Within the year, he'd worked his way down to E, echinacea. That seemed to bring some relief, and he stuck with it for a while, increasing the number of pills over time. But after a few months the pain returned in full force.

Fibromyalgia is so tricky to diagnose that the typical sufferer spends over five frustrating and demoralizing years shuffling from doctor to doctor, from specialty to specialty. Then, once diagnosed, there's usually another stretch of years as doctors and quasi-doctors experiment with a variety of uncertain treatments.

Delores, a thirty-eight-year-old mother of two, a fine artist from Tennessee, had a throat infection, fever, extreme tiredness, and severe pains in her hips, knees, and ankles. Her family doctor, who found nothing, sent her to an infectious-disease specialist. Finding nothing, he sent her to a rheumatologist, and she ultimately saw a neurosurgeon, who recommended a spinal operation. A good friend's sister, a nurse, told her she'd be crazy to go through such a delicate operation when none of the doctors was sure what was wrong. But Delores was taking antidepressants, prescription painkillers, and a few pills she could neither name nor tell you just what they helped with. After three years of running through a maze of white coats and enormous bills, she was feeling desperate.

The sister recommended that Delores first visit Nancy Selfridge, a family practitioner outside Madison, Wisconsin. Dr. Selfridge had just recently brought herself almost complete recovery from decades of fibromyalgia pain through a plan she'd devised after reading Dr. John E. Sarno's insights into back pain in his book *The Mindbody Prescription*. She taught Delores her program—and in two weeks Delores could use her knees, hips, and ankles without grimacing. She was able to quit one medication after another with her doctor's support.

Some think fibromyalgia is a new disorder. In truth, it's a constellation of symptoms that has been known since before the start of the twentieth century. Many in the media think fibromyalgia is what doctors call a status diagnosis, as trendy as getting your nose fixed or your tummy tucked. In truth, from 10 to 30 percent of all fibromyalgia sufferers are forced to survive on meager Social Security disability payments even though most of them are well-educated, intelligent, goal-oriented overachievers. Those virtues may in fact be their downfall, the prime mover or complicator that eventually triggers fibromyalgia.

Fibromyalgia is physical. It's not "all in your mind," despite what many doctors have told sufferers. It affects portions of the nervous system, including the centers that oversee our involuntary reactions such as heartbeat and breathing. It may start there, in what's known as the autonomic system—but many researchers now believe that it starts somewhere else and heads there. While affecting the autonomic portions of our nervous system, it sends physical signals all over the body, triggering pain and other symptoms.

The pain is involuntary—and it is real. It can be measured. Some of the biochemical changes it creates in the body and brain have been documented in lab experiments and reported in medical journals. One measurable physiological effect of fibromyalgia is that the body's most painful muscles and tissues receive less oxygen than normal.

If only doctors could manipulate this reckless set of biochemicals, we might be able to cure fibromyalgia. Many researchers are pursuing this approach. What complicates the search for a cure is that there are at least a hundred unique biochemical messengers, or neuropeptides, that facilitate communication between brain and body. They all can create physical effects, including pain. Almost all of the hundred were discovered in our bodies only within the past ten years. So researchers have a long road ahead.

FIBROMYALGIA: THE GREAT MASQUERADER

Patients who are diagnosed with fibromyalgia can often rattle off long lists of diagnoses they've received to explain their symptoms. These include irritable bowel syndrome (IBS), myofascial pain, tendonitis, fascitis, degenerative joint disease (DJD, also called osteoarthritis), and gastroesophageal reflux disease (GERD). Many researchers believe that all these separate disorders were and are initiated by the same process that got the fibromyalgia going. They're all symptoms of one illness.

One related illness is temporomandibular joint (TMJ) pain. A few years after fibromyalgia really clobbered Franklynn, but before his doctors diagnosed what ailed him, his jaws started feeling as if they were rusting shut. They made loud clicking noises and sometimes quit moving altogether. His dentist sent him to an orthodontist, who prescribed braces. Now, it's true that Frank had grown up with an overbite that your average grade-school kid calls "buck teeth," but given what we now know, it is likely that fibromyalgia, not the overbite, caused the jaw pain.

Fibromyalgia can occur at the same time you're fighting other illnesses or disabilities. It has been discovered in 10 to 40 percent of patients with lupus (systemic lupus erythematosus, or SLE), a disease with more macabre consequences than fibromyalgia. It's been discovered in 10 to 30 percent of patients with rheumatoid arthritis. Because of overlapping symptoms, however, many fibromyalgia patients have been first tested for both arthritis and lupus—and often misdiagnosed as having one or the other disease. They found out only much later that what they had was "only fibromyalgia."

Between 50 and 70 percent of patients with fibromyalgia have or have had diagnoses of chronic fatigue syndrome, IBS, migraine, or depression. Fibromyalgia shares with these other illnesses such symptoms as facial pain, paresthesia ("pins and needles," tingling or numbness of the limbs), urinary urgency, sicca symptoms (dry eyes, dry mouth), or premenstrual syndrome (PMS). This crazy quilt of interlocking symptoms and syndromes prompted one fibromyalgia physician and researcher to advise colleagues, "Little value exists in worrying whether a patient has fibromyalgia, chronic fatigue syndrome, or irritable bowel syndrome—or all three disorders."[4] To us, they now all seem to come from a common cause.

Some researchers lump myofascial pain syndrome and fibromyalgia together as one ailment; some separate the two. People who have one are likely to have the other. Myofascia refers to a type of tissue that covers our muscles. If the myofascia is irritated or mistreated, physically or chemically, it becomes very painful. The pain focuses at what are described as trigger points. They're different from the "tender points" that a doctor probes to confirm a fibromyalgia diagnosis, although both are a focus of pain. Researchers into fibromyalgia generally expect that if they find a cure for fibromyalgia, it will also be the cure for myofascial pain syndrome.

Many of fibromyalgia's symptoms are commonly found in people with clinical depression. In fact, antidepressant drugs have for a long time been used in an attempt to treat fibromyalgia. As a result, there's a legend that fibromyalgia sufferers tend to be depressives. Although 50 to 70 percent of fibromyalgia patients have had depression at some point in their lives, only 18 to 36 percent of fibromyalgia patients at any one time currently have major depression—about the same percentage of depressives found among rheumatoid arthritis sufferers, and very close to the percentage of major depression sufferers found in the so-called normal population.[5]

Which brings us back to a common complaint among fibromyalgia sufferers: fibro fog. As we mentioned, a few researchers dug into fibro fog and discovered, to everybody's surprise, that it can't be demonstrated to actually exist. The condition we feel as fibro fog may be the diminished mental skill that comes with untreated depression. Both depressed "normals" and depressed fibromyalgia patients go through bouts of fibro fog. In clinical tests, both groups show the same ability to remember, think, and process information.

Janet, a longtime fibromyalgia victim, tells how she couldn't even phone her husband at his office when she felt hit by fibro fog. Though she had a speed-dial phone programmed to reach his office, she'd freeze up after hitting that button. Her fingers refused to poke the digits for his extension in the right order. She knew the extension number, but the fog seemed to disconnect fingers and brain from each other.

Acceptance of the fog is so common among fibromyalgia patients that many of them simply assume they have to live with it as a semipermanent, unwelcome new part of their personalities. It's a self-defeating assumption, and it's not true.

While studying stress, Dr. Harvey Moldofsky, M.D., professor of sleep studies and psychiatry at the University of Toronto, subjected fibromyalgia study volunteers to a standard cognitive test. He gave the computerized test to individuals with fibromyalgia and to matched control subjects without fibromyalgia. Both groups were told to manage four different tasks they had to think about all at the same time.

Predictably, the fibromyalgia sufferers hated the experiment, while the controls liked it. But much to the surprise of the "foggy" fibros, who assumed they were doing poorly in the assigned tasks, they actually did them as well as the controls. They just took somewhat longer than the controls did.[6]

Did Dr. Moldofsky's research finding surprise you? It startled most of the fibromyalgia sufferers we monitor on support web sites and at support group meetings. It shocked some of them into rethinking whether there's truth in several other old wives' tales that they once thought were facts about fibromyalgia.

Fibro fog may be just one more of our brain's ways of coping with the pain and other life-darkening aspects of fibromyalgia. You can meditate or visualize your way out of it. (We introduce both techniques in a later chapter.) Or you can treat it like the tooth fairy and Easter bunny; did you notice how they quit coming around after you quit believing in them?

Fibromyalgia victims have believed in fibro fog for so long, it's a tough myth to kill. The first time Franklynn got a little ornery with Dr. Selfridge after she started treating him was when she told him that he wasn't having a memory problem at the moment, that he wasn't experiencing fibro fog, that there wasn't any such thing as fibro fog, and that he should quit using that term.

We worked hard to demolish the fibro fog myth for you just now so that you can give our mind-body technique your complete, unfogged attention. If this technique is to heal your fibromyalgia, you must let us work with your unfettered mind.

Chronic fatigue syndrome is another mystery condition of unknown origins and is still without a cure. It may be in some way related to "fibro fog," since it's found in a high percentage of fibromyalgia sufferers. Some doctors lump the two together and treat them together—but they still fail to find a cure for either one.

About one in five fibromyalgia patients we've met were victims of childhood abuse, sexual or otherwise. There's no doubt that this impacted severely on their souls. It may even have been the event (or series of events) that shoved the patient into fibromyalgia later in life. But many victims of abuse don't have fibromyalgia. So far nobody's conducted extensive research into the confluence, nor seriously studied whether abuse is one pathway to fibromyalgia. The good news is that it's probably not necessary to figure out what triggered fibromyalgia if it can be treated no matter how or when it started.

In the coming pages, we'll take the time to explain our treatment and to document the sources of our medical facts and opinions. We'll share with you the experiences of real people who healed within a few weeks, as well as those of individuals whose treatment dragged on for many months. The ones who quickly healed generally adopted the attitude "What the heck, can anything get worse?" They forced their minds into "obedience mode" so they could adhere to our assignments and schedules as faithfully and vigorously as they knew how.

The slow healers generally were those who clutched their skepticism as a security blanket. Like all of us, they'd tried "cures" before. They'd gotten their hopes up. They'd felt sorely dumped on when panaceas flopped. They were now going to "give this a try" but

CONDITION	PERCENTAGE OF FIBROMYALGIA SUFFERERS WITH THE COMPLAINT	PERCENTAGE OF "NORMALS" WITH THE COMPLAINT
Allergy	64.3%	40.8%
Balance problems	34.7%	10.6%
Bruxism (grinding teeth)	33.6%	14.2%
Chronic fatigue	72.0%	17.8%
Coccyx pain	35.9%	8.3%
Cold sores, frequent	28.5%	21.3%
Concentration problems	59.6%	14.3%
Constipation, chronic	40.2%	16.6%
Depression	64.4%	14.2%
Diarrhea, recurrent	34.5%	8.3%
Feet, burning	64.0%	18.3%
Fluid retention	44.6%	17.2%
Heat intolerance	42.4%	16.6%
Memory problems	53.2%	17.2%
Mitral valve prolapse (misshapen heart valve)	18.9%	5.3%
Muscle fatigue	65.2%	17.2%
Neck problem leading to surgery	15.3%	12.4%
Numbness, tingling	72.6%	14.8%
Palpitations of the heart	21.7%	7.8%

CONDITION	PERCENTAGE OF FIBROMYALGIA SUFFERERS WITH THE COMPLAINT	PERCENTAGE OF "NORMALS" WITH THE COMPLAINT
Pelvic pain	66.1%	23.1%
PMS	47.5%	23.1%
Restless legs (pins and needles)	49.1%	21.3%
Sciatica	53.2%	13.6%
Sexual dysfunction	66.6%	21.9%
Sinus problems	56.3%	33.1%
Sleep disorder: problems falling asleep	80.1%	23.7%
Sleep disorder: awakening during sleep	39.0%	36.7%
Stomach ulcer	18.2%	5.9%
Swollen glands	66.8%	7.1%
Tachycardia (heart rhythm anomalies)	50.4%	17.2%
Temporomandibular joint dysfunction (jaw spasms)	46.9%	8.1%
Tinnitus (ringing in ear)	50.5%	10.6%
Vertigo	40.2%	15.4%[7]

not throw themselves into the program. They hoped that way to limit the amount of dejection they'd feel in case this promise also soured for them.

Both Betsy and Anna approached our mind-body technique at this kind of arm's length, trying this and testing that—until suddenly some significant piece fell into place for them, the pain diminished dramatically, they took another big leap, and got well. We never could identify exactly what it was that shoved them over the top. Neither could they. But over the top they went, and they'll never be haunted by fibromyalgia again! You'll hear more about their experiences on Dr. Selfridge's program later in these pages.

FIBROMYALGIA'S MANY SYMPTOMS

It's getting easier all the time to say what fibromyalgia is not. Much harder is listing all the symptoms that a patient can suffer, and suffer in any combination. Pain is one pathway. Irritable bowel syndrome is another. Emotions are yet another. Nancy can still vividly recall her own bouts with low blood pressure (hypotension), so low she could faint nearly instantly. Cramps and vomiting were her unpleasant companions even during vacations.

But here, in alphabetical order, is what we can say with certainty are among the symptoms that fibromyalgia sufferers are prone to endure in greater numbers than the general population.

CONDITIONS THAT CAN AGGRAVATE FIBROMYALGIA SYMPTOMS

AGGRAVATOR	PERCENTAGE OF FIBROMYALGIA PATIENTS WHO REPORT THAT THIS MAKES THEIR CONDITION WORSE
Specific posture	81%
Weather change	80%
Specific kinds of lighting	78%
Noise	75%
Mental stress	75%
Physical stress	75%
Cold	47%
Repetitive motion	43%
Caffeine	35%
Heat	26%

What's important is not how many or how few symptoms on the list you relate to. What is important is the fact that we're here to help you make those symptoms disappear.

FIBROMYALGIA IS NOT ANOTHER "WOMAN'S DISEASE"

Xiao-Ming Tian, M.D., an authority on acupuncture and Chinese medicine, says that fibromyalgia was described in Chinese writings at least eight hundred years ago. The symptoms, causes, and patient outlook that were documented by ancient practitioners make up essentially the same lengthy list as today: muscle pain, widespread stiffness, fatigue, weakness, irritability. Even then, fibromyalgia flare-ups linked to weather factors such as cold, windy, and humid conditions, and to possible foreign bodies—including what we now call viruses and bacteria.[8] So little has changed in eight hundred years.

Close to 90 percent of known fibromyalgia sufferers are women. That alone virtually guarantees that most old-guard doctors—especially those who haven't kept up with medical literature—are going to pooh-pooh the pains, the sleeplessness, the hypersensitivity to sounds, smells, and touches. As a consequence, fibromyalgia sufferers shuffle from specialist to specialist, clinic to clinic, hearing one medical excuse after another.

Men with fibromyalgia are taken more seriously when they complain to doctors of pain. But that may not get them the right diagnosis either. When Franklynn started experiencing pain and losing his grip when he held a hammer, his two primary physicians were male. They teamed up to put him through test after test until he felt like a pincushion. They sent him to specialist after specialist until his insurance company quit paying for them. Never once did they wonder aloud if his body was misbehaving because of something in his head or because he wanted to goof off at his job. In fact, they warned him repeatedly that his demon was real and that he was not to think of it as psychosomatic, nerves, or some sign of character defect.

Eventually a savvy doctor did piece together the puzzle, figuring out that Franklynn had fibromyalgia. He admitted that there wasn't much they could do, but he consulted the medical literature and offered what was then the standard shot in the dark: prescriptions for antidepressant medication and regular exercise.

As a rule, only the wealthiest of female fibromyalgia victims we interviewed for this book received such kind, respectful treatment. The few who reached physicians like Dr. Selfridge were the lucky ones, because there are few physicians around the world who are treating fibromyalgia successfully.

Consider this: The physical conditions that make fibromyalgia so painful are more than likely to get worse over time. The longer you wait, the harder you are to treat. Don't delay getting the help you need. Let's get started—right now.

RELIEF IS AVAILABLE TODAY

If someone could figure out which one or more of the biochemical messengers that are responsible for pain was the rogue causing fibromyalgia, they might develop pills that guarantee coping or curing. However, there are at least a hundred neuropeptide chemicals in our bodies and many of them have to regenerate themselves precisely every twelve to sixteen hours in order to keep on working faultlessly. When they all work together, life feels good. When they clash, symptoms arise, and life becomes a living hell. Nobody's yet close to explaining which malfunctioning organ or chemical—alone or in combination—results in full-blown fibromyalgia. That's not surprising, since science still can't detail the precise neurochemical cascade that produces an embarrassed blush; all doctors can tell you is that it's "a selective blood-vessel dilation of the face and neck."

Fortunately for fibromyalgia sufferers, New York physician John E. Sarno, M.D., didn't wait around for biochemists to sort out which particular malfunctions create back pain before he developed a way to halt it in his patients. He found evidence that one major area of the brain, the limbic system, generates the chemicals whose effects can include turning on that awful pain. Armed with that insight and with exceptional sensitivity to his patients' concerns, Dr. Sarno devised a very effective way to treat back pain and related complaints. His method depended on his theory that the mind and body work together to produce the pain of what he calls tension myositis syndrome, or TMS. This theory was far enough outside medicine's mainstream that doctors weren't quick to duplicate his treatment, but word of his successes is spreading—and along with it go knowledge, understanding, and slow acceptance.

With the help of a colleague who knew of Dr. Sarno's work, Dr. Selfridge figured out how to apply Dr. Sarno's theory to understanding what was fueling her fibromyalgia. In four to five weeks her pain was almost a memory. Another four to five months later, her sleeping disorder was gone. Over time she rid herself of nearly all her fibromyalgia symptoms; she says she now feels 90 percent cured. She's a member of a busy medical group practice. She talks to fibromyalgia support groups. Hardest of all, she is the single mother of two teenage girls. And for fun, now that she feels mostly pain-free, she wins bike races and participates in triathlons.

Dr. Selfridge introduced her newfound method to patients, refining it according to their needs, and met with increasing success. To date she's successfully treated more than two hundred other fibromyalgia patients in her office—and uncounted others through her talks at seminars and meetings. Between 80 percent and 90 percent of Nancy's patients who are willing to try her treatment—which involves no pills and no operations—are now able to return to their normal lives, a result that's been duplicated anecdotally by other healthcare providers using Dr. Sarno's models in their approach to pain management.

Until now our method has mostly been used in clinics and controlled settings. With the help of committed patients who agreed to let us observe their progress in minute detail, we have fine-tuned our recommendations for self-directed recovery. We've come a long way in a brief time, and we can now ask you to join us in freedom from fibromyalgia.

Isn't it a bit unnerving that doctors call what
they do "practice"?

—George Carlin

EIGHT FIBROMYALGIA FABLES

Take it from Nancy Selfridge, M.D.: Doctors are
taught that it's wrong to say, "We don't know,"
so when they honestly don't know, they can say
some terrible things to patients. That's one
explanation for the many thoroughly demean-
ing, unscientific myths and rumors about fibromyalgia.

Let's explore the myths for what they are.
We want you to know as much as possible so
that you can make your own decisions as intelli-
gently as possible. Only then can you follow this
program wholeheartedly.

You see, it's nearly impossible to lick this
demon if you play by its rules. We want to show
you how to outwit it with a different set of
rules—ones that give you the advantage. They've

worked for hundreds of Nancy's patients and for thousands of patients we've learned about from other doctors. We hope you'll take some of our guidelines, tips, and schedules and make them your life's rules to achieve freedom from fibromyalgia. Again, we reiterate our hope that you'll also share this book with your medical practitioner—together you can form a more effective partnership to spread the word that real relief is available.

This is not another pop-the-pills program. It's not another wacky diet that quits ten minutes after the placebo effect wears off. We'll offer no "miraculous" supplements or "foolproof" jungle-grown cure-alls. We'll leave you with no side effects, no funny taste in your mouth. Our treatment plan is grounded in medical and scientific research. We've put our specific references in notes at the back of the book. We hope this book will help start a revolution in treating fibromyalgia effectively.

The treatment plan will require your participation—and a strong commitment to see it through. If you're not sure you're ready to stop being a victim, or if you're just sticking your toe in the water to see if maybe a frog who's really a prince will jump up to cure you, it's not likely to work well for you. But the more you know, and the faster you can accept what we explain here, the harder you can work at helping us help you—and the sooner you will be free from fibromyalgia's grip.

We must warn you—the treatment works at different speeds for different people. Nancy spent nearly five weeks curing herself of the pain and several more months correcting the sleep disorder that generally accompanies fibromyalgia. It took Franklynn only a week to get rid of his pains, but another three months to put his sleep disorder nearly to rest. He still fights occasional bouts with restless legs. But he too feels at least 90 percent improved.

As you work your way through the program, don't get concerned if you feel you need more time for a given step. What's important is to follow your body's instincts and to stay committed, starting now.

As we've told you, one of the most vital findings by mainstream medical research has been that for most people, fibromyalgia is not likely to just go away—in fact, for many people it only gets more severe and harder to treat over time. In a recent conversation, Dr. Sarno, the New York physician and medical school professor we met in Chapter 1, said that trying to cure fibromyalgia without facing up to its causes "is dangerous" because "new symptoms [can] occur."[9] Boston University researcher Maura Kennedy, M.D., studied fibromyalgia patients to find out which attributes best helped them beat this illness. Among her findings was that a "shorter duration of symptoms at the time of diagnosis" correlated with a better outcome.[10]

At the University of Alabama at Birmingham, Dr. James M. Mountz, M.D., Ph.D., and his colleagues ran hundreds of sophisticated whole-body imaging studies on fibromyalgia patients. Early in his published results, Dr. Mountz warned, "Researchers have begun to consider that . . . over time the pain may be maintained or exacerbated by functional alterations in critical regions of the brain and spinal cord which are involved in pain processing or pain inhibition."[11] In plain words, it's possible that fibromyalgia pain causes changes in your brain and spinal cord that themselves make the pain worse, make it last longer, or both.

THE LATEST RESEARCH SHOWS WHAT FIBROMYALGIA IS NOT

Anybody who's had fibromyalgia for a few years has probably read more than enough literature put out by various well-meaning organizations. Some of the information was based on then-current research, but few sources we've seen are up-to-date and completely free of fibromyalgia mythology. Unfortunately, corrections to old theories don't always get published and read. Let's separate the facts from the fiction.

FIBROMYALGIA FABLE #1: FIBROMYALGIA IS A FICTION DREAMED UP BY WELFARE FRAUDS

One of the most disheartening truths we face as we hunt through the medical literature for clues is that many reports start with the assumption that fibromyalgia is a malingerer's nonillness and fibromyalgia sufferers are welfare cheats, crying wolf and collecting checks. Welfare cheats? Do they really suppose that we want to stop going to work and instead sit around and enjoy excruciating pain?

A woman in Saskatoon, Saskatchewan, Canada, ran a successful small business despite her fibromyalgia. She knew that she needed to insure the company against all kinds of disasters, including the remote possibility of becoming too disabled to run the business. It's not that she was filing to collect disability payments due to her fibromyalgia; she wasn't disabled at all. But she was refused disability insurance because she had fibromyalgia.[12]

Harbor no doubts: Fibromyalgia is real. It is one of a group of related conditions that Dr. Sarno has been investigating for decades. It was added to the roll of known illnesses by the American College of Rheumatology and by the World Health Organization. The National Institutes of Health fund research into this enigma. Some U.S. insurance companies now pay fibromyalgia-related claims—though Dr. Selfridge's patients are finding claims for fibromyalgia disability increasingly difficult to pursue.

Don L. Goldenberg, M.D., a Newton, Massachusetts, physician and researcher, studied and compared hundreds of published research papers about fibromyalgia. In a lengthy journal article, he summed up his findings: "Most patients with FM [fibromyalgia] have had symptoms for five to seven years before a diagnosis is made. Once FM is diagnosed, the number of hospital admissions and health care use decreases."[13] In other words, once fibromyalgia sufferers know what they have, they ask for less medical attention, not more.

FIBROMYALGIA FABLE #2: FLAWED MUSCLES CAUSE FIBROMYALGIA

Among those doctors who do accept that fibromyalgia is an illness, a common misconception is that it's an illness of the muscles. It sounds logical because this ailment makes muscles nearly all over the body feel like they're on fire, being jabbed by pins, or being stretched to the breaking point. So for much of the past hundred years researchers have focused on the muscles of fibromyalgia sufferers in their search for a cause and a cure, and they've labeled the illness with muscle-oriented names such as fibrositis, muscular rheumatism, and, finally, fibromyalgia.

During this same hundred-year period, medical journals reported finding one muscular anomaly after another in fibromyalgia patients:

○ Muscle filaments with a "moth-eaten" appearance

○ Ragged red fibers, found in muscle biopsies

○ Separation of bundles of muscle fibers, called myo-fibril separation

○ Serrated or sarcolemmal muscle membranes

Over the years, the muscle "findings" have all been red herrings, misleading results not specific to fibro-myalgia—and definitely not helpful in determining the origin of sufferers' symptoms.

The century-long focus on muscles has not completely disappeared, but its heyday is past.[14] While fibromyalgia patients may tire and quit exercising sooner than so-called normal people, it's the pain that's to blame; a recent medical journal article reported that they do have normal muscles and normal muscle strength.[15]

FIBROMYALGIA FABLE #3: METABOLISM MALFUNCTION CAUSES FIBROMYALGIA

The next big myth about what causes fibromyalgia grew out of the muscle myth. It's that muscle metabolism is to blame. Metabolism is the biochemical process by which our cells consume energy-giving substances to produce raw materials for new cells or biochemical fuel to perform important jobs that our bodies need to do constantly if they are to stay healthy. If any one major energy generator were to malfunction, it could very well lead to excruciating pain as a muscle suffers an energy crisis. For decades, metabolic dysfunction was a favorite fibromyalgia theory. And sure enough, studies of fibromyalgia victims found:

○ Irregularities in mitochondria, the "energy factories" inside every living cell

○ Reduced levels of ATP, ADP, and AMP (adenosine triphosphate, adenosine diphosphate, and adenosine monophosphate, all essential to muscle function) in fibromyalgia patients' trapezius and other muscles

○ Reduced PCr (phosphocreatine, a metabolism by-product) in trapezius and other muscles

○ Abnormal levels of oxygen (too much or too little, depending on the researcher) in many of the muscles that were painful to move or touch

Unfortunately, many of the studies that found these effects suffered from a fundamental flaw that another researcher pointed out in 1998: comparing the muscles of fibromyalgia patients to the muscles of normal volunteers. It may sound like a logical thing to do, but Robert M. Bennett, M.D., an Oregon Health Sciences University researcher, points out that such studies do not factor in the reality that 80 percent of fibromyalgia patients are in lousy physical condition. Because of the pain, they don't use their muscles as freely as "normal" volunteers. Dr. Bennett was able to show that, in general, the same muscle and metabolism research findings would have resulted if the researchers had compared ordinary out-of-shape people to well-conditioned people.[16] The case for metabolic disorders has yet to be proven.

FIBROMYALGIA FABLE #4: FIBROMYALGIA IS CAUSED BY AN INFECTION SUCH AS EPSTEIN-BARR VIRUS OR LYME DISEASE

Medical researchers have hunted diligently for hidden microorganisms as the cause of fibromyalgia. They've already pointed a finger at the Epstein-Barr virus, commonly called EBV. EBV is a member of the herpes family of viruses to which many people are exposed at some point in their lives; among other things, viruses in this group cause chicken pox, infectious mononucleosis, herpes, and cold sores.

Fibromyalgia patients seem more likely than the average population to have reacted to herpes viruses with illness at least once. Franklynn, for example, had an unusual immunity as a child to chicken pox. In college, he twice came down with mononucleosis. Cold sores plagued him until he was about twenty-one. But whatever the reason for the frequency of herpes virus infections, nobody has yet been able to find proof that this virus causes fibromyalgia.

Lyme disease, a bacterial infection, presents an even greater paradox for fibromyalgia sufferers, their doctors, and researchers. Humans generally catch Lyme disease when bitten by the tiny deer tick, which can carry the Lyme bacterium. From 10 to 25 percent of patients with Lyme disease develop fibromyalgia within a few years after being apparently successfully treated for the infection. But despite a seeming connection, nobody has been able to document that this bacterium causes fibromyalgia.[17,18]

Edward, who's fifty-three years old now, spent six years bouncing between clinics like a pinball. One doctor treated his compression of three vertebrae from a motorcycle accident. Another prescribed antidepressant pills. A third medicated him for Lyme disease, since Edward had been bitten by a deer tick and gotten the traditional reddish bull's-eye-shaped blotches. But his painful symptoms would not let up. He says, "I went around to several more doctors who took a stab at curing me, but then a friend recommended Dr. Selfridge." She tested to make sure the Lyme disease had been successfully treated and found that his antibody levels were normal. She tested for the life-threatening diseases that mimic fibromyalgia symptoms. On his third visit, she could definitely say he had fibromyalgia.

The Lyme disease connection is more insidious than coincidental, at least from the vantage point of fibromyalgia sufferers. Between 25 and 50 percent of all patients who are referred to Lyme disease clinics—and treated with large doses of very unpleasant curatives—later prove not to have had it at all. They've had fibromyalgia, but it just wasn't properly diagnosed.[19]

While fibromyalgia is not contagious, studies suggest that certain genes may pass on a susceptibility among sufferers' children and grandchildren. So far there is no blood test to detect fibromyalgia or the gene (or genes) that may predispose to it. But there is a reasonably specific test that's used to support the diagnosis. In the test, a physician probes the eighteen most commonly sensitive zones on the fibromyalgia victim's body. If at least eleven of them are so painful that the patient can't stand even a gentle probe, the physician can be almost certain the problem is fibromyalgia.

FIBROMYALGIA FABLE #5: SLEEP DISTURBANCES, INCLUDING APNEA, CAUSE FIBROMYALGIA

Researchers have found many intriguing commonalities in the problems fibromyalgia sufferers have with sleep. In particular, we seem to spend less time in what's called stage 4 sleep. That's the sleep period when the body secretes most of the growth hormone that plays a role in repairing cells. Like Franklynn, men with fibromyalgia are more apt than women to have sleep apnea, a condition in which the sleeper stops breathing for anywhere from a few seconds to over a minute. But curing their sleep apnea does not relieve fibromyalgia's other physical symptoms.

One creative researcher, Dr. Harvey Moldofsky, deliberately disrupted stage 4 sleep among healthy volunteers. He found that they developed pains very similar to fibromyalgia. Dr. Moldofsky's subjects were luckier than us, however. After a couple of nights of good sleep, their fibromyalgia symptoms went away.[20]

Moldofsky also found that fibromyalgia patients have three times the number of spontaneous wakings during sleep as healthy people—arousals that happen for no apparent reason and last five or ten seconds before the patient goes back to sleep.

In a Swiss medical journal, a researcher questioned popular theories on what causes sleep loss in fibromyalgia sufferers. He suggested that maybe people with fibromyalgia have problems sleeping simply because they're in pain.[21] Makes sense to us!

Physicians have placed a lot of emphasis on treating the sleep problems—maybe because there are pills for that. But while the pills have helped some of us sleep better, they rarely relieve other symptoms.

FIBROMYALGIA FABLE #6: INJURIES CAUSE FIBROMYALGIA

Some people with fibromyalgia believe the disease originated with an accident, most often a car accident. In nearly every other way, however, these fibromyalgia sufferers resemble the rest of us. Little research has been done on the subject, but one study did find that compared to those with fibromyalgia not linked to any specific trauma, those suffering from post-traumatic fibromyalgia were

- More sensitive to cold

- Less sensitive to noise

- Less sensitive to light

- Less sensitive to mental stress

- More sensitive to repetitive-motion disorders

- More likely to have sciatica

- Less likely to have pelvic pain or sexual dysfunction

- Less likely to have a rapid heartbeat (known as tachycardia)

- More likely to have "restless legs" or a pins-and-needles sensation[22]

Nobody yet knows why.

FIBROMYALGIA FABLE #7: IT'S AN IMMUNE DISORDER

Over the past ten years we've seen several flurries of excitement as researchers seemed to have found something in the immune system that causes or cures fibromyalgia. It certainly sounds like a reasonable place to dig for clues. But so far no immune system link has been positively identified.

This is not to say that the immune system is totally uninvolved with the development of fibromyalgia. Almost without exception, fibromyalgia patients' bloodstreams carry a number of antibodies not found in other adults. Antibodies are large protein molecules secreted by B-lymphocytes (white blood cells). Each antibody is designed specifically to attack one foreign body displaying a specific characteristic, known as an antigen. But these antibodies do not appear to be more than one group of players among many in fibromyalgia's development. They're as likely to be an effect of the disorder as they are to be a cause.

FIBROMYALGIA FABLE #8: IT'S ALL IN YOUR HEAD

As each body-oriented hypothesis has failed to be proven, more and more research has turned to our central nervous systems and brains, which certainly play a major role in fibromyalgia. First, scientists focused their attention on how nerves transmit pain. That's a particularly complicated function. It involves both electrical and chemical signal processing. The chemicals involved include (but are not limited to)

○ Body-building organic chemicals known as amino acids (such as tryptophan)

○ Neurotransmitters, which are information-transmitting chemicals (such as L-dopa and serotonin)

○ Prostaglandins (hormones active in information responses, sex organs, and other functions)

○ Nitrous oxide (laughing gas), a building block of elements of the central nervous system

○ Mineral ions, which are chemically and electrically active forms of minerals such as iron, selenium, and calcium

○ Natural painkillers known as endorphins

Early on, researchers seeking clues in the brain focused on serotonin, a major biochemical that helps to regulate signals passed between various parts of our body, including the brain. Many studies found reduced levels of serotonin in fibromyalgia patients. Since other studies had reported reduced serotonin levels in depressives, many physicians began to prescribe antidepressant medications routinely to fibromyalgia victims. Some of us who've had fibromyalgia now think of Thanksgiving as our holiday, because turkey is chock-full of tryptophan—and tryptophan metabolizes in the body to form serotonin. Unfortunately, though antidepressant drugs and over-the-counter

St. John's wort and 5HTP all increase levels of serotonin, all have failed to eliminate fibromyalgia's symptoms.

One of the next major brain-oriented clues researchers studied was an elusive neurotransmitter labeled substance P. The P stands for *pain*, because this little messenger appears to be vital in transmitting pain signals throughout the body. It works by increasing the size and number of pain-sensitive nervous system cells called neurons. Fibromyalgia sufferers have double or triple the amount of substance P compared to a "normal" population. (Ulf von Euler, a Swedish biochemist who first identified the existence of substance P in 1931, shared a Nobel prize for its discovery in 1970. However, it was Susan Leeman, a Harvard biochemist, who finally identified and explained its complex chemistry in 1971—though Harvard denied her tenure and she has yet to make the trip to Stockholm.)[23]

Perhaps in an attempt to counter the effects of increased levels of the pain-promoting substance P in our systems, fibromyalgia patients tend to have increased blood levels of a natural painkiller known as dynorphin A. It's one of many natural opium-like chemicals that the body makes. These painkillers' generic name is endorphins (if you're in the United States) or enkephalins (if you're British).[24] Dr. Selfridge often wonders if such natural painkillers might explain why she felt foggy and fatigued some days with her fibromyalgia. Postoperative Demerol, a narcotic, gave her a similar experience.

As we write this book, medical researchers are investigating one brain chemical and electrical circuit after another, hoping to find the magic bullet to rid us of fibromyalgia, but with every gain in scope and specificity comes an increase in complexity. We'll devote the next chapter to bringing you up-to-date about the body signals that appear to fuel fibromyalgia and the countersignals that we can initiate to defuse the demon. The fact that this messaging system is not centered only in the brain impacts mightily on how we reach freedom from fibromyalgia.

From here until the end of this book we're going to spend precious little time on causes or symptoms or aggravations. We'll put you on your way to freedom from fibromyalgia using a program that has worked for us and for thousands of others like us.

Rheumatologists need to vocalize in exponential repetitive fashion, "We don't know what we are talking about."

—Sean F. Hamilton, M.D., F.R.C.P.C.

3 FIBROMYALGIA 101:

WHAT IT IS

If anybody tells you that fibromyalgia is "all in your head" or incorrectly uses the term *psychosomatic* to suggest that you're afflicted with mental pathology and your physical symptoms are imagined or unreal, that person doesn't understand the last two decades' advances in medical science. Most doctors are trying to drop the emotionally charged term *psychosomatic* as it's been used in the past. Now much of modern medical science focuses on the interdependence between the head—or, more properly, the brain—and the nervous system, on what is called the mind-body connection.

Fibromyalgia is best approached and treated as a condition headquartered in our central nervous system, but the latest research tells us that the system's activities—both normal and unusual—are not confined to the brain and the network of interconnected nerves. It's now clear that the immune system and endocrine system both play key roles in the central nervous system's communication of data, requests, and orders to different parts of the body. The endocrine system generates hormones and other active chemicals such as insulin, estrogen, and serotonin far from the brain, in organs such as the pancreas, liver, spleen, and gonads. The immune system generates in the spleen, bone marrow, and elsewhere the cells that respond to foreign substances in our body, such as bacteria and viruses.

There's another new wrinkle. You may have learned in school that the brain-and-nerve network operates by using electrical impulses that leap from neuron to neuron to send our body's messages hither and yon. Biochemist Candace Pert, when she was at the National Institutes of Health, and other basic researchers have identified a rich array of chemicals that are involved in sending and receiving mental, emotional, and body-related messages. In fact, we now know that the biochemical system carries more messages than the electrical messengers of our nervous system, and the messages generally are more critical to our overall health.

These messenger chemicals are often called neuro-peptides or neurotransmitters. More recently, however, many researchers have been dropping the neuro-, as it's pretty clear that these messenger molecules move through more parts of the body than just the brain, spine, and nerves, and are generated outside these central areas too.

We're now going to simplify and explain all three systems that are part of our central nervous system: the classic nervous system, the immune system, and the endocrine system. If you know how they work, you'll better understand where fibromyalgia comes from. That will help you start taming it—fast.

THE CLASSIC NERVOUS SYSTEM

The classic nervous system described in most textbooks was assumed to include only the brain, spine, and networked nerves. It's a major element in the body parts and functions that generate fibromyalgia. Various scientists divide its components in different ways. We'll use the simplest way.

The *autonomic function center* is the part of the brain that handles all "autopilot" functions such as pumping blood, breathing, digesting food, and regulating our body temperature. It is often called the brainstem, hindbrain, or reptilian brain. (*Reptilian* refers to its evolutionary past; it was added to the evolving nervous system tools during an age populated mostly by reptiles.)

The *limbic system* was probably the next brain system added through evolution. Physically it encircles the brainstem. It creates the chemicals of emotion and may also play a role in memory. Among the brain structures incorporated in the limbic system are the recently discovered amygdala (two almond-shaped structures inside the brain, about one inch from each ear), the hippocampus, and the limbic cortex.

The *cerebral cortex*, built into the front of our brain, handles reasoning and logical communications among the body systems, among other functions. Within the evolutionary process, this is the newest of the nervous system's communication centers.[25]

Here's how they work together while we're in, say, a Jamaican craft market. When we see something we really like, or when we get angry at an overaggressive "higgler" from whom we're trying to purchase a trinket, our limbic system leaps into action to create a sense of excitement or annoyance. When we've narrowed our purchases down, the cerebral cortex figures out the currency exchange rate, so we know that a J$1,200 painting costs about $30 in U.S. currency. The whole time, our autonomic systems are keeping our hearts beating, our lungs breathing, and our skin sweating in response to the rise in body temperature caused by our activities and the hot Jamaican sun.

During most of the twentieth century, scientists believed that the brain communicated to other parts of the body over an elaborate electrical system. The mighty brain, our electrical nerve center, sat atop the major regional signal wire, the spinal column. Smaller bunches of nerve wires snaked out from the spine to major parts of the body. Nerves do pass electrical signals, but we now know this is a small part of the signaling that takes place between the brain and other parts of the body.

Scientists had one major leap to make before they could fully understand the classic nervous system. There is a physical gap, called a synaptic cleft, between neurons, or nerve cells. At first nobody could explain how the body's low-amperage, low-voltage current jumped over that gap to deliver its message. Dr. Pert and co-researcher Dr. Miles Herkenham were among the people who discovered what really happens.

It turns out that when one of those tiny electrical charges reaches the end of one neuron, it sets off a chemical explosion that hurls dozens of specialized molecules, known as neuropeptides, across the gap and toward the receptors of the surrounding neurons. These neuropeptide molecules complete the message delivery process.

But Pert, Herkenham, and others learned that these messenger molecules are not localized only in parts of the body rich in nerve impulse transmission points (called synapses). By the time they'd remapped the way our central nervous system works, Herkenham estimated that less than 2 percent of brain-centered communication actually takes place via the electrical synapse system. The rest relies directly on messenger molecules—smart chemicals.[26]

THE CHEMICAL SYSTEM ENHANCES THE ELECTRICAL NERVOUS SYSTEM

There is now no doubt that the overwhelming majority of messages communicated through your body—probably 80 percent or more—move via smart chemical molecules. There is also no doubt that modern medicine has been excruciatingly slow to learn and use this chemical messenger system in diagnosis and treatment, and that slowness impacts particularly badly on those of us with fibromyalgia. Physicians (and the rest of us alike) really cannot understand how we get fibromyalgia or how to cure it unless they are willing to learn at least the fundamentals of how the chemical nervous system works.

In the 1970s medical science thought there were only two neuropeptides: acetylcholine and norepinephrine. Because of an accidental discovery—that acetylcholine sets a switch "on" and norepinephrine sets it "off"—early researchers thought that neurotransmitter chemicals were just an extension of the electrical system, helping electricity flow (when the neuron was "on") and not flow (when it was "off").

But neuropeptides are much more sophisticated than that. The brain's neurons bring messages to the areas where these chemical molecules are manufactured. When an area gets a message, the right peptide races through the body, often replicating itself in other body tissues also capable of manufacturing the peptide and hence its message is delivered with greater speed and efficiency. It doesn't stop until every essential part of the body has received the message—even places where there are no electrical neurons.

When researchers discovered the neuropeptide dopamine, it was at first suspected as a culprit in schizophrenia.

Then they found the pain-killing peptides known as endorphins or enkephalins.

Researchers demonstrated how these smart molecules work even before they'd identified their chemical makeup and given them names. One famous experiment tapped a bit of spinal fluid from a sleeping cat and injected it into a wide-awake cat. That cat soon fell asleep. After the first cat woke up, they tapped more spinal fluid, injected it into the still-sleeping cat, and that cat woke up too. The experiment proved that in cats, neuropeptides carried brain-fed signals to go to sleep or wake up.[27] Additional research showed that the same mechanisms are part of human central nervous systems.[28] But it took a long time before medical doctors understood the experiments' implications.

By now, investigators have uncovered at least one hundred more peptides, and there are probably others hiding in our bodies to be discovered. Each peptide has a unique shape, chemical structure, and task or set of tasks to accomplish by carrying precise messages throughout our bodies. The peptides can't just bump into random parts of your body and give off their signals. To work, each peptide has to find a cell with a specifically shaped receptor into which it can fit snugly and remain fastened semipermanently. This pairing with a matching receptor is often pictured as a key fitting into a lock.

Your cell walls are quite smooth except for the receptors "glued" onto their outside walls. Each receptor is "sticky" because its outermost molecule is open-ended, just waiting for an appropriate peptide to find and fit into it. When a fit is made, it forms a complete, very stable molecule. More than that, the peptide that has just fit into the receptor can be thought of as carrying a message from the brain or from another organ; the message changes some aspect of the cell's function.

Under an electron microscope you can actually see this process and follow individual peptides as they head directly for their target receptors. It's a bit like watching sperm cells wiggle their way toward egg cells, except hundreds of times faster. And unlike sperm, which all head toward one egg cell, neuropeptides fan out with their message toward hundreds or thousands of receptor cells.

The brain is not only the sender of important messages that tell key parts of the body how to behave. It too is rich with receptors, so it can receive enormous numbers of simultaneous messages about how various parts of the body are behaving. It can get these messages because other systems, such as the immune system, generate peptides too.

What parts of the body are high enough in the pecking order to be bothering the mighty brain with messages? Well, just about every other part that exists, but especially the immune and endocrine systems.[29] Ironically, ancient Greek philosophers were not terribly far off the mark when they argued that the liver was the center of our nervous system, and the Renaissance scientists who believed our spleen was central to our well-being were just about as correct as "modern" scientists who think the brain is the only key to everything our body does. We now know that the liver (an important part of the endocrine system) and the spleen (part of the immune system) are particularly active members of the team of body parts that labor long and hard to keep us healthy and happy.

Researchers finally understand that the central nervous system is fundamentally chemical. Messenger molecules stream into the nervous system from the pancreas, kidneys, pituitary, intestines, and reproductive organs. For example, the hormone prolactin is a messenger molecule that signals breasts to produce milk shortly after other hormones have finished assisting in giving birth.[30]

These findings require us to spend a little time reexamining the immune and endocrine aspects of the central nervous system, and to pinpoint their role in causing and curing fibromyalgia.

A CLOSER LOOK AT THE IMMUNE SYSTEM

Older medical texts paint the immune system as a nearly self-contained, self-controlled body defense system. But new findings tell us that neuropeptides travel into and out of it. In truth, our bodies are not made up of separate, unconnected systems. The spleen, bone marrow, lymph nodes, and white blood cells—key players in the old classic model of human immune systems—produce neuropeptides in addition to their immune-specific secretions. They're equipped to send messages to that other defense line, the central nervous system. In fact, around 1982 researchers started finding that just about every messenger molecule in the central nervous system has matching receptors on key immune cells. Take the monocyte, for example, a key white blood cell, or lymphocyte, that talks to other lymphocytes with names such as B cell, T cell, and killer cell. Its cell walls are rich with sticky receptor sites designed to receive specific matching neuropeptides.[31]

It turns out that nearly every key immune cell can generate and send throughout the body nearly every known peptide. Nearly every key immune cell can receive and interpret nearly every known peptide. The immune system is so intimately tied in with the brain and central nervous system that it makes good sense to treat it as one component of the central nervous system.[32]

Treating the central nervous system holistically, researchers have found new jobs that its components perform. Some of those tasks may create or prevent fibromyalgia symptoms. Given these facts, some doctors and biochemists have now started to drop their imagined fences between the body and the brain, or body and mind. Most recently they've linked the immune system to something once considered totally outside the realm of medical science—the emotions.

Specific emotions, we now know, all trigger specific neuropeptides, and some of these peptides signal the immune system to start performing some of its jobs. Dr. Pert explains, "These emotion-affecting peptides, then, actually appear to control the routing and migration of monocytes [white blood cells], which are very pivotal to the overall health of the organism."[33] She adds, "The immune cells are making the same chemicals that we conceive of as controlling mood in the brain. So immune cells not only control the tissue integrity of the body, but they also manufacture information chemicals that can regulate mood or emotion. This is yet another instance of the two-way communication between brain and body."[34]

What Dr. Pert says is crucial: Your emotions have direct power over your immune system—and your immune system has direct power over your emotions.

Knowing how to use that connection is vital in curing fibromyalgia.

A CLOSER LOOK AT THE ENDOCRINE SYSTEM

A similar link exists between the classic nervous system, the immune system, and the endocrine system, the organs that generate hormones and other beneficial chemicals used by our bodies. These include the kidneys, pancreas, gallbladder, liver, thyroid, gonads, and pituitary gland. All send and receive messages to and from the brain and immune system.[35]

We now know that organs once thought to have a monopoly on the production of certain chemicals are not the only source of those chemicals. For example, the pancreas is the body's largest producer of insulin, but the brain makes it too. The messenger molecules transferon and CCK, once considered tools only of the brain and the electrical aspects of the central nervous system, are now known to be made elsewhere as well and can be received by receptors outside the brain. Whenever the brain wants to signal you that your stomach is full, it secretes CCK. It goes directly to the stomach, as you'd expect, but when replicated into more messenger molecules, it also lands on receptors all along the intestinal tract to keep it working. It signals the gallbladder to get ready to release stored bile, a chemical that digests fat. It signals the spleen—the chemical factory of the immune system—that digestion is in progress, so it shouldn't waste energy by starting to attack foreign objects such as the meal you just ate.[36]

In the endocrine system, emotions generate cascades of messenger molecules. We already learned about one such group of messenger molecules, the neuropeptides called endorphins that are the brain and body's built-in painkillers. When you deliberately change your rate or depth of breathing—as do practitioners of yoga, meditation, and the Lamaze childbirth method—the flood of messenger molecules that your brainstem releases includes endorphins.

We know of one hormone that specifically malfunctions in fibromyalgia: growth hormone. It regulates the regeneration and growth of nerve cells. The connection between it and fibromyalgia was identified and reported in medical journals over a decade ago, but again, nobody yet understands the full picture.[37]

WHERE DOES THE BODY END AND THE BRAIN START? AND WHERE IS THE MIND?

We've seen how the brain, the immune system, and the endocrine systems are intimately connected—to such an extent that we've come to understand them as one system. As Dr. Elmer Green, a Mayo Clinic physician who pioneered biofeedback for treatment of disease, puts it, "Every change in the physiological state is accompanied by an appropriate change in the mental emotional state, conscious or unconscious, and conversely, every change in the mental emotional state, conscious or unconscious, is accompanied by an appropriate change in the physiological state."[38]

Do you need tangible proof from everyday life? How about butterflies in your stomach? Fear and timidity cause real physical turmoil within our stomachs as the hormones and digestive enzymes kick up unpleasant chemicals. Or goose bumps? Excitement releases chemicals that stimulate the pilo-erection muscles around hair follicles, making bumps we can see and touch.

The gifted motivational speaker and physician Dr. Deepak Chopra sums up what we've just learned this way: "It has now been absolutely proved that the same neuro-chemicals influence the whole bodymind. Everything is interconnected at the level of the neuropeptide; therefore, to separate these areas is simply bad science."[39] The body and mind are inextricably interlinked and interdependent to such a degree that we must consider the whole of mental and physical and emotional body functions as one unified system. The study of this unified system has a new name, psychoneuroimmunology. If it's new to you that the body and mind are unified, not separate, welcome to the forefront of modern medicine, finally treating the person as a whole instead of part by part.

State-of-the-art knowledge about fibromyalgia and its treatment comes from researchers who have abandoned the old checkerboard approach to medicine: one square for gastroenterologists, others for pulmonary specialists, gynecologists, psychiatrists, neurologists, virologists, and so on. The lines dividing the checkerboard seem to be what has limited the scope and amount of care any traditional specialist can offer those of us with fibromyalgia.

"Life is intelligence riding on chemicals," Dr. Chopra says.[40] We like this summation so well, we put it on plaques to hang on our office walls. It reminds us to think of our bodies as self-managed, integrated systems instead of as awkward composites of discrete physical, electrical, and chemical machines.

Dr. Chopra asks skeptics to explain why, when a cold virus is sprayed into the noses of eight volunteers, only one of them, on average, comes down with a cold, and the immune systems in the other seven wipe out the virus easily.[41] His answer: Seven minds are healthy and keep the immune cells healthy. One mind, unhealthy or distracted or angry, interferes with normal immune response. The unhappy but predictable result is a cold. Dr. Chopra says that he must "spend much of my time just talking, trying to get people not to be so convinced by their disease . . . As long as the patient is convinced by his symptoms, he is caught up in a reality where 'being sick' is the dominant input."[42]

John Sarno is professor of clinical rehabilitation medicine at New York University School of Medicine and a practicing physician. In the 1970s he began applying mind-body medicine to treat patients. At first he experimented on his own migraines, then with patients who had migraines. He found that those who knew there was some kind of emotional tension involved got better, while those who rejected the connection did not.[43] His keen insights into the mind-body connection have filled three books, and he's become celebrated for treating patients with ailments as diverse as back pain and fibromyalgia. He tells us he finds fibromyalgia patients are among the hardest to help.

Dr. Sarno, along with a growing number of scientists and health providers, believes that the areas of the brain responsible for emotion are directly involved in generating not just body effects such as the blush, but all sorts of musculoskeletal pain. He uncovered evidence that pain could be produced by emotion-generated chemicals, even if the emotion was not consciously acknowledged, and he concluded that many of the patients in his practice weren't responding to traditional treatment for pain because they hadn't received the proper diagnosis. In short, they were being treated for the wrong ailment.

Applying what was already known about the workings of the mind, Dr. Sarno suspected that the unconscious emotions responsible for his recalcitrant patients' pain generation were the strong emotions, such as rage, that were considered unacceptable in polite society. When asked, many of his patients named stressors or unpleasant circumstances that could be influencing their pain. But Dr. Sarno knew that pain was not directly caused by these external events; rather, the patients' experiences produced emotions that in turn stimulated the production of specific neurochemicals, which resulted in specific bodily changes felt as pain. Patients who accepted this new explanation for their pain got strong relief almost immediately. Those who said they doubted that emotions were the root of their physical suffering did not improve.

Dr. Sarno calls pain generated in this specific way tension myositis syndrome, or TMS. In three breakthrough books he elaborates on these ideas, which have helped more than ten thousand patients lose their pain under his care. He emphasizes that knowing, understanding, and finally accepting the fact that emotion is causing one's pain is sometimes sufficient to eradicate or significantly relieve it. In his treatment, he documents patients' symptoms and, if they have TMS, explains how it begins in emotion. He invites them to lectures in which TMS is more thoroughly explained. If they aren't better after the lectures, they can attend small support-session discussions.

Dr. Sarno does not distinguish between TMS and fibromyalgia by calling them different names. We see it a little differently. We think that fibromyalgia is all of TMS all at one time in just one body, and we continue to use the term fibromyalgia because patients and colleagues are familiar with it. Still, we are grateful to Dr. Sarno for finally helping us understand this heretofore baffling syndrome.

Dr. Selfridge was introduced to Dr. Sarno's work by a sympathetic colleague. She read his book *The Mindbody Prescription* and recognized the logic of his words. For years she had felt intuitively that her own fibromyalgia pain and its other symptoms had to be originating in the brain. Here, at last, was a scientific explanation! But unlike so many of Dr. Sarno's patients with back pain, she did not get better all at once—nor did most of her patients. She was discovering that most, if not all, fibromyalgia sufferers have characteristics that complicate their response to Dr. Sarno's treatment approach.

Dr. Sarno had already noticed that TMS patients tend to be perfectionists and to be "good people." Dr. Selfridge soon learned that most of her fibromyalgia patients were also sensitive types. They were not wimps, but they responded more strongly than other patients to the environment. They were more sensitive to noises and sounds, to smells and tastes, to changes in temperature, to the texture of their clothing. Most important, they were more intuitive, noticing and responding more to the emotions of people around them. Dr. Selfridge's observations were supported by the research of Elaine Aron, Ph.D. In her book *The Highly Sensitive Person*, Aron reports that with or without psychological problems, a very sensitive person has more physical pain than other people.

As we've noted, the medical literature suggests that more fibromyalgia patients have had severe psychological trauma, such as sexual abuse, than the general population. Dr. Sarno says that 40 to 60 percent of his fibromyalgia patients required psychotherapy to improve. But Dr. Selfridge finds a much smaller percentage. In her busy family practice, Dr. Selfridge took care of many women who had been raped or molested but did not have fibromyalgia. On the other hand, she's helped many people with fibromyalgia who had no remarkable psychological history. So she rejects psychological trauma as the common denominator that keeps some fibromyalgia patients from responding completely to mind-body treatment, and is slower to suggest psychotherapy.

Dr. Selfridge admits she's highly sensitive. While she was applying Dr. Sarno's treatment to her own symptoms, she was sometimes distracted or just feeling overwhelmed by daily living. It wasn't easy to reflect on the emotions that might be instigating her fibromyalgia. She recognized that she had to structure more downtime to accomplish this goal. To help her focus, she adapted some of the tools she had learned in psychotherapy. Franklynn, by nature much more creative, added variations that helped him recover with remarkable speed. While helping Franklynn treat his fibromyalgia, his partner, Judi, learned the mind-body technique—and in two sessions she cured her own painful esophageal acid reflux, which had resisted all medications for a year. Like back pain, it was a straightforward mind-body symptom.

Understanding that some people may be resistant to the very new, Dr. Selfridge still offers her own fibromyalgia patients a choice: tests and pills, or this more generally successful method of coaxing our brains into curing us. Most patients now choose the mind-body method, which this book will guide you through even if you live many miles from a doctor who can teach it to you in person. In these pages, we will teach you how to do what it takes to make your own body, your own brain, your own mind, and your own hectic life stop generating fibromyalgia—the pain, the lousy sleep, the nervous legs, the whole awful thing.

We offer you these tested tools knowing that they'll help many of you come to know more complete relief from your symptoms than you ever believed possible. And we credit Dr. Sarno with giving us the key to our insights. His books are essential reading for anyone interested in mind-body treatment.

THE TRIGGERS THAT BRING ON FIBROMYALGIA

For sensitive people like us, it helps to understand some of the triggers that can contribute to fibromyalgia. It starts with an emotion such as shame or anger or rage. It's not the usual you-didn't-pick-up-your-socks kind of anger, or even the gosh-I-don't-know-why-I-lost-my-job anger. It's deep anger that you may not have ever let yourself see as anger, anger that's never been vented, never been recognized as anger. It's the primitive fight-or-flight anger that psychiatrists call narcissistic rage; it's probably programmed into all humans' genes, and it is *unconscious*, or beyond our ability to consciously recognize it.

You, like us, may have learned very young—as a little person living with your giant-like parents—that it was unsafe to express rage, grief, shame, and other strong feelings, whatever the cause, that it was safer to hold them in. If you were physically or verbally abused as a child, that could cause even greater shame and rage.

Perhaps you grew up amidst tensions too over-whelming for your sensitive nervous system, shoving you relentlessly toward the impossible goal of being perfect or being very, very good all the time. Perhaps just the tensions common in all families seemed to have more of an effect on you, while your caretakers never helped you learn to tend to your emotional needs. Now you've had a significant loss—of a loved one, a job, status, or income—or a significant emotional shakeup, such as a car accident. Society's message, enforced by the 80 percent who are not sensitive types, is that you must just buck up and get on with your life. But we sensitive types need time to process the pain, to recover emotionally.

It's the emotional impact of the loss or the physical trauma, the unconscious anger or other deep emotion it generates, combined with society's message to get on with your life that may stimulate the production of chemicals that create fibromyalgia symptoms. You've been given a genetic container for your deep emotions; it's well accepted that at times, circumstances cause the container to overflow. We believe that when this happens, the dread sensitive people like you have of expressing—or even feeling—your deep-seated emotions becomes greater than your dread of physical pain. So your mind, brain, and body conspire to generate a constellation of real physical symptoms out of the raw, repressed emotion, to create a distraction from the chaotic and painful experience deep within.

Dr. Selfridge found it difficult to believe that any part of her, even her unconscious, would choose physical over emotional pain—until she remembered the months surrounding her divorce, a period so emotionally charged that it almost incapacitated her. Though some of her symptoms were at their worst when her marriage was exploding, her emotional pain was so great that she can easily say now that she would readily choose any physical pain over that degree of emotional pain any day. Now, remarkably, she discovered that if you convince your body that you know what's going on— that it's turning unrecognized anger, grief, or shame into distracting physical pain by flooding your body with peptides—your unified mind-body system will quit generating those automatic responses. It will expel your fibromyalgia. Your thoughts and beliefs, now changed into neurochemical messages, will signal the body to stop making symptoms.

Once you learn and practice this, it'll be as easy as sneezing, only much more rewarding.

Does it sound too easy? It *is* that simple! Without waiting until science knows exactly how the triggers do their dirty work, fibromyalgia sufferers can bring themselves back to health.

STRESS AND FIBROMYALGIA

Fibromyalgia sufferers are more sensitive to stress than the general population. Some of us can barely tolerate loud noise, unpleasant odors, excessive exercise, or hot or cold weather. Although Franklynn enjoys eating fish, when he had fibromyalgia he couldn't stand the smell of it cooking.

Looking back, Dr. Selfridge can point to the various stages of fibromyalgia as it crept insidiously into her life. It started in high school with irritable bowel syndrome (IBS), one of the illness's disguises, as she worked like a demon to pull the grades to get into the "right" college. In college, on the stress-filled pre-med track, her lower back, neck, and shoulders started aching. Fibromyalgia hit harder during her medical residency, when she was stressed out, exhausted, and unable to control any aspect of her life. Looking back, it's not surprising that her fibromyalgia symptoms all got worse, and that she got new symptoms: whole-body pain, sleeping problems, fibro fog. Adding to her stress, she got married that year—and relaxed just long enough for a thirty-six-hour honeymoon. She was a walking fibromyalgia machine, filled with emotions that churned out fibromyalgia-making chemicals.

Treating deep-seated stress such as Dr. Selfridge's is complicated by the fact that it is responsible for physical changes, behavioral adaptations, the release of hormones, and more. A June 1998 paper in *The American Journal of the Medical Sciences* by Dr. Leslie J. Crofford, a rheumatologist and fibromyalgia researcher at the University of Michigan, demonstrated tangibly that stress increases the number and severity of fibromyalgia symptoms.[44] Dr. Crofford also reported that two brain-body communication channels don't function properly in fibromyalgia patients: the channel linking the brain's hypothalamus to the body's HPA neuroendocrine axis (consisting of the pituitary and adrenal glands) and the channel linking the hypothalamus to the HPG neuro-endocrine axis (consisting of the pituitary gland and the ovaries or testes). Since the reproductive organs generate and use sex hormones, this communication fault in the HPG neuroendocrine axis may explain why fibro-myalgia attacks so many more women than men. Some of the irregularities in chemical communication between brain and body that are implicated in fibromyalgia may also be related to premenstrual syndrome, irritable bladder, and chronic headaches.

The following diagram shows how Dr. Crofford believes our genes, physical makeup, and stresses under-lie the events that can trigger fibromyalgia.

Diagram modeled after an earlier medical journal diagram prepared by Dr. Leslie J. Crofford showing the progression of physical and emotional conditions that can lead to fibromyalgia.

Causes of variations in neuro-endocrine responses to stress

Genes   Childhood stress
Gender   Adult stress

Causes of vulnerability to stress in fibromyalgia

Unhealthy or extreme responses to acute stress
         Emotional
         Psychological
Unhealthy or extreme responses to ongoing stress
         Emotional
         Psychological

Trigger that brings on the fibromyalgia

Trauma or degeneration due to things such as . . .
         Whiplash
         Repetitive motion injury
         Osteoarthritis
Inflammation due to things such as . . .
         Rheumatoid arthritis
         Systematic lupus
Virus or bacteria infection due to things such as . . .
         Lyme disease
         Viral illness
Psychological stress
Hormonal stress

FIBROMYALGIA

Fibromyalgia is not a condition that comes and goes. Once it starts, it keeps its grip on the body even though symptoms may fade in and out. Every time symptoms return, they get more severe—and you may be clobbered by new symptoms as well. Events with significant emotional impact get "downloaded" into your brain's limbic system, where they leave a permanent record. At the age of twenty, most people have not yet downloaded enough junk to make fibromyalgia rear its ugly head. Add some more emotional or physical stress to a sensitive nervous system, and by thirty you may have accumulated enough to bring on fibromyalgia full force. You can't run. You can't hide. You probably can't erase your body's chemical and physiological changes.

Here's how Dr. Pert explains what you're up against:

> The body is the unconscious mind! Repressed traumas caused by overwhelming emotion can be stored in a body part, thereafter affecting our ability to feel that part or even move it. The new work suggests there are almost infinite pathways for the conscious mind to access—and modify—the unconscious mind and the body.[45]

Dr. Selfridge tells patients to think of our book's fibro-beating program as "better living through better mind-body chemistry." Every emotion generates chemistry. Our mind is not separate from our body. So, she counsels, attitude is almost everything.

Let's start there.

PART

2

TOOLS TO BATTLE

FIBROMYALGIA

I can complain that my rosebush has thorns, or
marvel at the thorn bush with its beautiful
flowers. It's all up to me.

—Anonymous
(found on a fibromyalgia support web site)

PUT YOUR NEW 4

KNOWLEDGE TO WORK

Every emotion and thought generates chemical
activity within your brain and the rest of your
body. Your body and brain can transmute
repressed negative emotions into pain symptoms.
We know that this process is part of the human
makeup and occurs in almost everyone—after all,
what else is a tension headache? But your sensitive nervous system probably exaggerates the
process. So to stop your symptoms, we need to
help you flood your brain and body with positive, happy emotions, to generate as many "up"
chemicals as possible to combat the pain-causing
messengers.

You may have noticed already that your
symptoms seem less intense when you're
relaxed and happy, and worse when you are sad,

mad, or tense. Cultivating the very chemistry of positive emotions will help clear the way for the specific thinking that will move you from fibromyalgia to freedom.

MAKING LOTS OF HAPPY CHEMICALS WILL GET YOU WELL SOON

While we're working with you to achieve freedom from fibromyalgia, help us help you. Think pleasant thoughts. Read books and view programs that are positive, happy, and upbeat. Until you reach freedom from fibromyalgia, try to avoid situations that may turn dismal on you. Try to avoid dismal people. This isn't Pollyannaish, mindless peppiness. Remaining positive is biologically critical to your recovery.

If you start thinking gloomy thoughts, change them using inspirational and motivational tapes or books, which you can find at libraries, bookstores, and even greeting-card shops. Many uplifting motivational speakers hold forth on radio and TV. If you're homebound, much of the legwork can be done online or on the phone if somebody can pick up books and tapes for you.

Dr. Selfridge puts it like this: "Look for blue sky instead of blue clouds." She tells patients and fellow practitioners about the study that Dr. Robert Bennett performed on two closely matched groups of fibromyalgia sufferers at the University of Washington Medical Center. Despite both groups reporting similar symptoms, the group whose members had a positive attitude about life felt they did well. The group that had a negative attitude felt they did poorly. In other words, the patients got from their treatment just about what they expected they'd get. That's why it's important, whenever you pick up this book or start your quiet time or assert your needs, to think of it as another step in getting well.

Betsy and Anna, two Wisconsin women who suffered from fibromyalgia, began their healing program by deliberately surrounding themselves with happy, uplifting little books of sayings, advice, poems, pictures—whatever it took. Here's one example they liked by an anonymous poet:

> DON'T QUIT
> *Success is failure turned inside out,*
> *The silver tint of the clouds of doubt,*
> *And you never can tell how close you are,*
> *It may be near when it seems so far.*
> *So stick to the fight when you're hardest hit.*
> *It's when things seem worst that you mustn't quit!*

At every fibromyalgia meeting they took part in, they started and ended with a cheerful reading. They had to cope with half the energy and twice the pain that humans are supposed to have—and without their positive attitude, they might never have made it to freedom from fibromyalgia. But they did.

Don't dismiss this apparently simple mechanism. When you're in pain, you might want to lash out at someone who quotes at you, "Laughter is the best medicine." But it worked for Betsy and Anna. It's worked for others. It will work for you.

Following our guidelines, Betsy and Anna also carefully restructured important parts of their lives. Betsy, for example, gave up a high-paying job in management, where the stress and long hours proved to be too much. She couldn't juggle meeting the job's demands and fighting her fibromyalgia. Recognizing that job stress was a significant emotional fibromyalgia trigger, she took another, lower-paying job for which she was significantly overskilled. It's a life change that greatly helped her lick fibromyalgia.

There are two additional consequences of Betsy's decision. First, cutting back on work hours and stress freed up precious time and energy for the critical task of healing herself. Second, deciding that her most important job was to heal served notice that she was putting her mind and body—her whole self—into the effort.

In time, Betsy may go back to something like her previous job, now that she's recovered from fibromyalgia and learned to prevent a relapse. She probably will be able to handle it again and not get a recurrence of fibromyalgia.

Anna couldn't change her situation as easily. Loving and caring by nature, once a week she spent an afternoon with a friend who had a serious heart condition. As her friend's health worsened, Anna's fibromyalgia pain did too. Then Anna learned that to heal fibromyalgia, she had to keep activating happy chemicals in her brain and to focus nearly exclusively on getting well. Recognizing that this important relationship was a significant emotional trigger, that catering to her friend's low spirits was jeopardizing her steps toward health, she began arranging cheerful lunches with her friend at a popular restaurant and trips to see upbeat movies. She avoided situations that invited long, gloomy talks.

It worked. Now Anna's fibromyalgia is a soon-to-be-distant memory.

You too can help yourself heal fibromyalgia. Let's take the first step right now.

STEP 1: DECIDE THAT YOU'RE READY TO BE WELL

Your combination of sensitivity and symptoms means that you need structured guidance to focus on the emotions causing your illness. If the program alone doesn't work, you may benefit from the specific guidance of a psychotherapist to help you uncover and cope with hidden emotional trauma. But first try our program.

Strange as it may seem, some readers may decide—consciously or unconsciously—that they aren't ready yet to take the steps to start getting well. We need to address that problem right here and now. Take the time to examine your own mind. Dig into the deepest recesses of your conscious and unconscious feelings and ask yourself, "Do I absolutely, positively want to get well, totally well?"

What in the world could get in the way of your wanting to feel well?

How about litigation? Are you suing someone because of your fibromyalgia or something related to it? Will getting well jeopardize your lawsuit? Would you rather put your energies toward the chance of money from litigation instead of toward freedom from fibromyalgia? Be brutally honest with yourself. Dr. Sarno and others who treat chronic pain patients all report that patients in litigation don't get better. Patients must invest a lot of emotion in winning such a lawsuit, and they need to prove they're "not well" to win.

What about Social Security disability? Are you collecting payments now? Or have you applied in the hope of starting to receive those checks? After you're well, the checks may stop. Think about what you'll live on, how you'll support yourself or your family. Make sure your attraction to health is stronger than anything.

If you get well and return to work, would you be returning to work that you love? There's little motivation to get well if your healthy future holds a pressure cooker of a job or another emotionally toxic environment.

How are your personal relationships doing? How strongly are they based on your suffering from fibromyalgia? Think again about your answers. Look more closely at each one of your personal relationships—with spouse, parents, children, friends. Do some of the family or friends you count on seem to respond most warmly when you're in pain or most tired? Are they most loving when you're feeling most helpless or hopeless? Do you think they'll be less devoted after you're well? Will they have to learn how to live with you in a different relationship? Will they want to make the effort? Will the cheerful, chipper, alert, pain-free you be able to bond with them anew? Might you lose any of them? Might they begin to expect more, maybe too much, of you?

You are not alone. It's common for newly treated fibromyalgia sufferers to weave new kinds of relationships with family and friends. You may want to use the following Relationship Planner now to help you sort out your relationships into those that might go sour as you gain freedom from fibromyalgia, those you might want to give special attention to as you get well, and those that you may want to kiss good-bye because they were built on pain, not pleasure. In general, the people who knew you well before fibromyalgia got its tentacles around you are most likely to remember the old you and welcome you back. But watch out for the dangerous exceptions, the people who thrive *because* you're not thriving, even if they claim to have your best interests in mind.

At one fibromyalgia seminar, a nurse revealed just how far you may have to go. Her sister had fibromyalgia. She herself was suffering from a close relative of fibromyalgia, chronic fatigue syndrome. They'd both spent years of frustrating visits to one doctor after another, swallowing one nonmiraculous "miracle herb" after another, all the while leaning for comfort on the local chronic pain support group.

Eventually both sisters reached the same conclusion. They decided it was time to step back and examine more deeply their painful lives—to try whatever had a chance to make them well. After several weeks of soul-searching, they realized that their support group could be part of the problem. They concluded that it was supporting their pain, not their quest for a cure. They dropped out of the group and lost touch with most members, and things started looking up. They both began feeling better and found new energy to heal themselves.

You may have to make the same kind of hard-nosed decision to ensure that you can move unimpeded down the path to freedom from fibromyalgia.

Relationship Planner

Which relationships are likely to support my freedom from fibromyalgia?

Instructions: Begin filling in this chart now or during Week One (see Chapter 10). Use a pencil—as life gets better, you may change your mind! Besides helping to analyze relationships, this worksheet aims to help you overcome indecisiveness, something that hampers many fibromyalgia sufferers. So avoid "maybe" answers as much as possible. Once a week, take out this chart and work no more than ten minutes trying to eliminate the maybes.

STEP 2: SCHEDULE TIME FOR YOUR TREATMENT

Before you can start your healing treatments, you need to set aside healing time. Make sure that you consider this treatment time important. Make a deep commitment in advance, not haphazardly as you go along. Plan now for time to do all the homework we assign you, all the writing and thinking and similar exercise we've created. Plan now to fill in all the forms carefully and thoughtfully, and to spend time focusing on searching for the emotions causing your fibromyalgia. Since sufferers often feel very busy, very stressed, very short on time, it's important to schedule each week of fibromyalgia work in advance. Only then can you make sure that all these important tasks get done.

We've divided up your homework into five separate units. In Chapter 11 there's a formal schedule for you to fill in. We think of each period as one week long, but remember, we're flexible. If you find that a week's worth of tasks saps too much energy, stretch the unit to two weeks, ten days, or whatever works better for you. But before you decide on a more leisurely schedule, examine closely whether your feeling of busyness is real or just part of your old strategy for coping with fibromyalgia. Consider how big a dent fibromyalgia—the real enemy—has made in your normal routine. Do you deserve less quality time than your demon?

COLUMN 1 PEOPLE WHO INTERACT WITH YOU REGULARLY	COLUMN 2 NAME OF PERSON	COLUMN 3 IS RELATIONSHIP POSITIVE?	COLUMN 4 RELATIONSHIP STARTED BEFORE FM? AFTER FM?
Spouse or live-in partner	_____	◯ Yes ◯ No ◯ Maybe	◯ Pre ◯ Post
Family (parents, children, siblings)	_____	◯ Yes ◯ No ◯ Maybe	◯ Pre ◯ Post
	_____	◯ Yes ◯ No ◯ Maybe	◯ Pre ◯ Post
	_____	◯ Yes ◯ No ◯ Maybe	◯ Pre ◯ Post
Friends/ neighbors	_____	◯ Yes ◯ No ◯ Maybe	◯ Pre ◯ Post
	_____	◯ Yes ◯ No ◯ Maybe	◯ Pre ◯ Post
Co-workers	_____	◯ Yes ◯ No ◯ Maybe	◯ Pre ◯ Post
	_____	◯ Yes ◯ No ◯ Maybe	◯ Pre ◯ Post
Others— shopkeepers, bankers, brokers, etc. (add more lines if needed)	_____	◯ Yes ◯ No ◯ Maybe	◯ Pre ◯ Post
	_____	◯ Yes ◯ No ◯ Maybe	◯ Pre ◯ Post

COLUMN 5	COLUMN 6	COLUMN 7	COLUMN 8
IS THIS RELATIONSHIP LIKELY TO SURVIVE MY HEALING?	IS THE RESULT IN COLUMN 5 OKAY WITH ME?	NOTES ON WHAT'S NEEDED TO FIX OR ELIMINATE THIS RELATIONSHIP	HAVE I FIXED THE RELATIONSHIP?
○ Yes ○ No ○ Maybe	○ Yes ○ No ○ Maybe	_____	○ Yes ○ No ○ Maybe
○ Yes ○ No ○ Maybe	○ Yes ○ No ○ Maybe	_____	○ Yes ○ No ○ Maybe
○ Yes ○ No ○ Maybe	○ Yes ○ No ○ Maybe	_____	○ Yes ○ No ○ Maybe
○ Yes ○ No ○ Maybe	○ Yes ○ No ○ Maybe	_____	○ Yes ○ No ○ Maybe
○ Yes ○ No ○ Maybe	○ Yes ○ No ○ Maybe	_____	○ Yes ○ No ○ Maybe
○ Yes ○ No ○ Maybe	○ Yes ○ No ○ Maybe	_____	○ Yes ○ No ○ Maybe
○ Yes ○ No ○ Maybe	○ Yes ○ No ○ Maybe	_____	○ Yes ○ No ○ Maybe
○ Yes ○ No ○ Maybe	○ Yes ○ No ○ Maybe	_____	○ Yes ○ No ○ Maybe
○ Yes ○ No ○ Maybe	○ Yes ○ No ○ Maybe	_____	○ Yes ○ No ○ Maybe
○ Yes ○ No ○ Maybe	○ Yes ○ No ○ Maybe	_____	○ Yes ○ No ○ Maybe

For now, don't let yourself schedule anything more than two weeks per treatment unit—and schedule to work at that rate only after you've paused a day to reflect on your priorities. Stretching out the required work over two or more weeks might not result in the kind of treatment intensity that forces fibromyalgia out of your system. Don't worry just yet that you won't be able to finish the scheduled work in time. Later we'll help you figure out what to do in case that becomes a reality.

STEP 3: READ THIS WHOLE BOOK FIRST

Before you begin any of the other exercises starting in Chapter 10, first read this book cover to cover. Read and enjoy the success stories. You can learn from them and adapt others' methods to your needs.

Absorb the overall message. Start thinking about the process we'll lead you through in the next few weeks. Focus on the end, where you'll be free of fibromyalgia. But study the steps, advice, and tips all along the way that will help you win your freedom. Realize that all the exercises exist to reinforce your understanding and acceptance that *unconscious emotions cause your symptoms*. We are, as Dr. Sarno says, helping you to meet those emotions at the door of the unconscious. You will be calling your mind/body on the carpet for trying to distract you with physical symptoms!

When Dr. Selfridge introduced Franklynn to Dr. Sarno's book, explaining that she'd been able to adapt its techniques to treat her fibromyalgia, Franklynn had to read the book twice before he was sure he understood it fully. He felt he was fighting a major fibro fog at the time. We suggest that if you do not now fully understand the mind-body process causing your symptoms, you pause to read Dr. Sarno's book before you start any exercises. We'll also ask you to reread this book along the way. Bear with us.

STEP 4: DISCUSS YOUR PLANNED TREATMENT PROGRAM WITH FAMILY AND FRIENDS

To succeed in getting well, it is important that you focus a major portion of your energy for at least five weeks on actively healing yourself. Because of your sensitivity and the fibromyalgia sufferer's typical sense of being overwhelmed, you will require solitude during your healing sessions. If you have commitments to people who might otherwise intrude into your solitude, discuss your plans with them. Share your schedule with them. Tell them how important this undertaking is to you. Ask them for their support, love, friendship, cooperation, and understanding. If they give it freely, great! You're already way ahead of others who have to fight for the space in which to get better. Just be sure that those who agree to cooperate really do stick to their good intentions—and plan to remind them if they forget.

You can't be Ms. Nice Gal or Mr. Nice Guy now. You need time, space, and concentration. They are essential. Tell family and friends right up front and in plain words that you are counting on them—that your healing depends on their full acceptance of your program.

If after all of your preparations, personal relationships still intrude, deal with them immediately. Try to figure out and fix what's wrong, what's keeping you from getting the rehabilitation time you need. Look again to see if—and how—those actions by others may be triggering the emotions feeding your fibromyalgia. Do the actions betray a fear of their being unable to relate as well to your better, stronger self? Encourage their trust in your continuing relationship by reminding them of your goal.

But deal firmly with each intrusion so that it doesn't happen again.

Simplify your life as much as you need to. Your family and friends may protest, but none of them can possibly know the degree of simplification you need now and maybe forever.

Betsy found the simplification she needed most for her treatment to work. "I always got upset doing dishes, but I never before thought to use paper plates! I do now, even though I know it's considered environmentally wasteful. I figured out that in ten years, I may throw away the equivalent of one tree." Betsy got the idea of paper plates from one of the inspirational and self-help books that she buys, borrows, and reads by the dozen, all part of staying focused on the positives in her life.

Keep your own eyes peeled for ways to simplify the demands on you.

If necessary, arrange to move your sessions to where you're less likely to be disturbed. Go to a parent's, friend's, or relative's home. Go to a camp. Go to a motel. Go to a library. Go wherever you have to in order to devote full attention to the program for two sessions a day for a minimum of five weeks.

Clergy often have resources to help you find a quiet place. Also check out resources that may be available through fibromyalgia support groups, Arthritis Foundation chapters, and women's support networks. Ask local hospitals' women's or educational departments whether they have or can recommend a quiet place.

Janelle had fibromyalgia for eleven years before being diagnosed correctly. Harold, her husband, scoffed at the diagnosis. He urged her to go on the pill-and-exercise treatment recommended by traditional doctors. When Janelle heard that Dr. Selfridge was scheduled to speak to a nearby support group in a couple of weeks, she asked Harold to go with her. There, right after Dr. Selfridge explained her mind-body technique, stressing the importance that a change in thinking plays in successful treatment, Harold turned to Janelle. "See?" he said smugly. "You just have to change your attitude." Janelle suddenly realized that part of her problem in dealing with fibromyalgia had been decades of living in a relationship that gave her no pleasure, only pain. Sure enough, after separating from Harold, her mind became free to triumph over fibromyalgia.

We hope that you don't think we're unfairly picking on family members. But the truth is, family members do often contribute to the emotions that give you fibromyalgia symptoms. You'll need to factor in whether they and their actions generate fibromyalgia-producing chemicals inside you. If so, you must either get them to help you or create some distance from them to minimize the emotional aggravations and distractions they create. Discuss what you've learned about cause and treatment. Explain what you now know about how fibromyalgia starts. Once they understand how the chemicals generated by emotion create pain and other symptoms, they may be willing and able to help you focus on these emotions. Knowing that they're in your corner will speed your success.

STEP 5: GIVE YOUR FIBROMYALGIA SYMPTOMS A NAME

Once you've made the decision to get well, give your fibromyalgia a name so that you can call it up to confront it. Do that by graphically describing it in your own terms. Be sure the name paints a vivid picture in your mind.

Dr. Selfridge thinks of her fibromyalgia as a child having a tantrum, demanding attention in an inappropriate way. Mothers and fathers can easily relate to that image. Franklynn calls it his demon. Cynthia sees fibromyalgia as a dingy-looking rock. (We'll tell you later what she does to that rock.)

Why pick a name you can visualize? After you achieve freedom from fibromyalgia, you may undergo a minor setback, perhaps caused by injury or exceptional amounts of stress. Having a name with which to quickly conjure it up will help you to look back and remember how bad it used to be. Looking back at a graphic personification of your old illness makes it faster and easier to send the demon, the tantrum-throwing child, the whatever-you-call-it running out of your life again.

Now that you have a name for your fibromyalgia, write it in at the top of the Historical Record of My Key Milestones chart in Chapter 8 and on the inside cover of the journal you'll be keeping.

STEP 6: FIND A "FIBRO SPOT" THAT SIGNALS TROUBLE

Take heart. You *can* heal. While we don't know if our techniques correct the biochemistry or the misdirected nervous system signals that cause fibromyalgia, what the exercises seem to do, in a medically sound, long-term way, is to force your brain to stop sending pain, drowsiness, and all those other awful symptoms to the rest of your body.

All the exercises we'll guide you through are there to help you structure the way you reflect on rage and other negative emotions. Remember, the emotions that cause fibromyalgia are unconscious and are likely to remain that way. It is the purposeful search for them and acceptance that they are the source of your pain that appears to interrupt the biochemistry that causes your symptoms.

But temporary setbacks are part of the process, and we must learn to recognize these as well. So after you complete the program, it's important for you to stay alert and attentive to signals that your body is building up for another attack. Generally, they show up in the form of subtle pains. Most often those subtle pains emerge in a "fibro spot," a favorite location in your body. Consider it a warning. When your "fibro spot" alarm goes off, focus not on the pain but on assuring your brain that you know what it's up to in creating the pain. Has something triggered your anger? Is something unresolved? Did your old angers collect to create more fibromyalgia? Once you're free of the symptoms, you'll know how to deal with a harmful emotion. Do it then and there, before it gets stored away or added to others. Consider the signal an opportunity to search for any rage, anger, shame, grief, or other emotion that's been submerged. At the sound of the alarm, dig it up and deal with it directly. Simply tell your brain, "Hey, you can't fool me any longer. I know you're trying to turn some hidden emotion into fibromyalgia." That confrontation alone usually works wonders.

Don't expect to know yet how to deal with pain you may experience in the future. You may not be able to identify your trouble signals until you're fully freed from fibromyalgia. We just want you to know about it now so that you can see what's at the end of your journey.

Franklynn's "fibro spot" is his left biceps. He can be working out at the health club, spinning and leaping and prancing and kicking, when suddenly he feels that special kind of warning pain in the very middle of his left biceps. Because he knows from experience that he can beat back his demon, he keeps working out while, at the same time, starting to look for its cause. When the demon strikes during aerobics, it's generally because he's still angry that, say, his partner didn't hustle out the door fast enough when they were leaving home half an hour ago. He acknowledges to himself that this frustration could be a trigger for the deep rage that creates his fibromyalgia symptoms. And just making that mental connection is enough to short-circuit his brain's fibromyalgia circuits. Defeated, the pain recedes fast.

Recently Franklynn was giving a speech to several hundred CPAs in Cincinnati when his biceps called, "Alert! Alert!" He knew immediately what it stemmed from. He'd forgotten to bring the remote-control button for his computerized slide show and was angry with himself for not being better organized. He also knew what to do about it: nothing, since making the connection between the equipment difficulty and his anger had already fixed the problem. Within four or five seconds, his mind was 100 percent back on telling the CPAs how to automate aspects of their work; he hadn't given his fibromyalgia a toehold.

Only very rarely now does the pain ever move beyond Franklynn's biceps. But it can happen. Alarms can still go off anytime, anywhere.

Note that Franklynn's anger at the Cincinnati meeting was not *external*; it didn't come from interaction with anybody else. But whether he was angry at himself, at the busy schedule he'd accepted, or at the organizers who had scheduled him to speak too early in the morning, it wasn't in the least important to find or point a finger at the actual source of the anger. When he felt the onset of fibro-spot pain, he knew that the pain (and most of its other symptoms) had been cooked up deep inside his brain. And he knew from a year's experience of freedom from fibromyalgia that all he had to do was acknowledge to his brain that he had experienced anger. Once he took that step, his brain backed off and the fibromyalgia quit again. Like the incantations spoken by shamans in many societies, acknowledging his demon worked what seems like magic.

You may want to keep an eagle eye out for angers that you cause yourself. A majority of fibromyalgia sufferers tend to be perfectionists, or what Dr. Sarno calls "goodists" (needing to do the right thing for other people, yet tending to feel uncomfortable when doing the right thing for themselves). These two personality types—often both are found in the same person—can be setups for fibromyalgia and other chronic-pain experiences. Nobody can go through life being perfect all the time, and it's human to wish that others did as much for you as you do for them. A bout of perfectionism or goodism might start a fibro spot aching. Be alert!

Betsy gets a big fibro spot in the middle of her back. It's so real that her acupuncturist found it one day. Without knowing anything at all about the Sarno technique, he said, "There's lots of anger there." Betsy noticed that she holds her breath when that fibromyalgia pain starts creeping up on her. She found she can fight it away just by acknowledging it's there and then taking several deep breaths.

Dr. Selfridge doesn't have just one fibro spot. She jumps to attention at any pain she notices anywhere. So one day she got fooled. Starting to hurt on her drive to work, she asked herself, "I wonder what big, bad, hairy emotion is so incredibly important right now that it's distracting me with this pain." And though she thought hard, she couldn't find any anger, guilt, or shame right then in her life—not with her kids, not with the idiot drivers on the road, not even with herself. The technique rarely brings to the surface any repressed source of anger. Nonetheless, just focusing on the mind usually chases away her pain.

But this day it was worse by the time she got to work, and she couldn't understand why. She was exasperated, because it was the first time her fibromyalgia-healing reflexes had failed her. And the discomfort climbed steadily. Pretty soon she was lying on her office floor—in excruciating pain. Finally her assistant came in and suggested that maybe this pain came from only her body. They ran some lab tests and, sure enough, found a strictly physical cause. Later that morning Nancy passed a kidney stone.

It's an important lesson. Part of freedom from fibromyalgia is recognizing that from time to time you will experience physically rooted aches and pains. You'll recognize them as the ones that don't respond to the techniques that chased your fibromyalgia away. You'll feel the joy of growing old in good health, but you'll still be subject to the occasional physical complaints that can happen to any older person. In a way, this is reassuring. Your fibro-fighting techniques will only work for emotionally generated pain. You won't misinterpret the pain of organic disease, such as a tumor, because pure body pain will not respond.

STEP 7: DON'T CHANGE TOO MUCH TOO FAST

Do you find it exciting to be launching your ship toward a shore where, only weeks from now, you will land free of pain, fatigue, and all those other dehumanizing fibromyalgia symptoms? Don't get so excited that you toss out your medications and ignore your regular schedule. It could add extra difficulty to the task of accomplishing this most important life change. At this beginning stage you probably have no idea which medications were helping what condition, which meds your body—and your brain—really needs or wants. Dumping them prematurely will complicate your life needlessly and may actually delay your reaching freedom from fibromyalgia. Doing so without a doctor's okay could be harmful, so never stop taking any medication without checking first with your doctor. There's plenty of time to drop them after you've reached freedom from fibromyalgia and gotten the go-ahead from your M.D.

Also, for now, stick close to the schedule that has made your life livable. Don't stress yourself out by over-scheduling, even for fun times. There's plenty of time to add happy activities to your life. Spend the upcoming five weeks convincing your brain and body that you are boss. Relearn what it feels like to be in control.

STEP 8: PLAN FOR YOUR WELLNESS

Here's our prescription for getting in the right mood to succeed at what's ahead: Plan now what you're going to do with some of the extra happy hours you'll have in your life just a few weeks from today. After years of putting it off, Dr. Selfridge finally found the energy to sell her old house and move her family to the center of town so that she wouldn't have to car-pool all the time. After years of procrastination, Franklynn—a born tinkerer until fibromyalgia pain took over—finally designed and built a three-season room from an old back porch. Cynthia loved to run before fibromyalgia laid her low. After examining her, Dr. Selfridge pre-dicted, "You will run again in a month." And sure enough, the minute Cynthia felt that she was "over the hump," she slipped on her running shoes and headed out to run and run and run.

In Week One you'll be asked to fill in the form below (*My Past, Present, and Fibromyalgia-Free Future*). It will help you put your planning into black and white, but look it over right now to start your mind thinking about qualitative assessments of you life. Don't be afraid to think big. You can do anything your mind sets you to!

STEP 9: GO FOR IT!

My Past, Present, and Fibromyalgia-Free Future

There are four parts, and you'll find them prescheduled for use at different times during Week One. Don't fill in all four parts in the same session. Stick to our schedule. When you've finished the first three parts, our schedule will direct you to go to the fourth part and compile the results. We'll tell you what to do with those results in later chapters so we don't influence your answers now.

1. Use ink. Don't change your answers.
2. Don't compare your answers in the first three parts of this form until told to do so.
3. There is a new set of instructions after the end of part C.

ASSESSMENT OF LIFE BEFORE FIBROMYALGIA

Answer on a scale of 0–10 (10 = most, highest, best)

1. My overall satisfaction with the last significant job I had before fibromyalgia set in: _____

2. My assessment of *how well equipped I was* to perform that job before fibromyalgia set in: _____

3. My assessment of *how well I actually did* perform that job before fibromyalgia set in: _____

4. How satisfying was the salary from that job? _____

5. My expectations of advancement at that job were: _____

6. How important was it for me to fulfill family obligations before fibromyalgia set in? _____

7. How do I rate the degree to which I did fulfill family obligations before fibromyalgia set in? _____

8. The amount of pleasure I *expected* from my family before fibromyalgia set in: _____

9. The amount of *actual* pleasure I derived from my family before fibromyalgia set in: _____

10. The degree of pain I *expected* from my family (0=most pain) before fibromyalgia set in: _____

11. The degree of pain *actually received* from my family (0=most pain) before fibromyalgia set in: _____

12. The amount of fun I *expected to have* on my/our last vacation before fibromyalgia set in: _____

13. The amount of fun I *actually had* on my/our last vacation before fibromyalgia set in: _____

14. The degree of satisfaction I *expected* on my/our last vacation before fibromyalgia set in: _____

(continued)

ASSESSMENT OF LIFE BEFORE FIBROMYALGIA

Answer on a scale of 0–10 (10 = most, highest, best)

15. The degree of satisfaction I *actually had* on my/our
    last vacation before fibromyalgia set in: _____

16. The amount of fun I *expected to have* on my/our next
    vacation before fibromyalgia set in: _____

17. Before fibromyalgia, the approximate number of days
    between times when I thought about a vacation idea: _____

18. The approximate number of weeks after my/our last
    vacation that fibromyalgia really set in: _____

19. My energy level before fibromyalgia set in: _____

20. Overall, I'd rate the energy level of the average per-
    son to be: _____

21. Overall, I'd rate my satisfaction with my life before
    fibromyalgia: _____

22. Overall, I'd rate the satisfaction of the average per-
    son with their life: _____

23. Overall, before fibromyalgia I'd rate disappointment
    and pain in my life (0=high, 10=low):   _____

24. Overall, I rate disappointment and pain in the life of
    an average person (0=high, 10=low):   _____

ASSESSMENT OF LIFE RIGHT NOW

Answer on a scale of 0–10 (10 = most, highest, best)

1. My overall satisfaction with any job I have: (if you have no job but want one, enter 0) _____

2. My assessment of *how well I am able to* perform that job: (if you have no job but want one, enter 0) _____

3. My assessment of *how well I actually do* perform that job: (if you have no job but want one, enter 0) _____

4. How satisfying is the salary from this job? (if you have no job but want one, enter 0) _____

5. My expectations of advancement at this job are: (if you have no job but want one, enter 0) _____

6. How important is it for me to fulfill family obligations now? _____

7. How do I rate the degree to which I fulfill family obligations now? _____

8. The amount of pleasure I *expect* from my family now: _____

9. The amount of *actual* pleasure I derive from my family now: _____

10. The degree of pain I *expect* from my family (0=most pain) now: _____

11. The degree of pain *actually received* from my family (0=most pain) now: _____

12. The amount of fun I *expected to have* on my/our last vacation: _____

13. The amount of fun I *actually had* on my/our last vacation: _____

14. The degree of satisfaction I *expected to have* on my/our last vacation: _____

(continued)

ASSESSMENT OF LIFE RIGHT NOW

Answer on a scale of 0–10 (10 = most, highest, best)

15. The degree of satisfaction I *actually had* on my/our last vacation: _____

16. The amount of fun I *expect to have* on my/our next vacation: _____

17. The approximate number of days since I last thought about a vacation idea: _____

18. The approximate number of weeks since my/our last vacation: _____

19. My energy level now is: _____

20. Overall, I'd rate the energy level of the average person to be: _____

21. Overall, I'd rate my satisfaction with my life now: _____

22. Overall, I'd rate the satisfaction of the average person with their life: _____

23. Overall, I'd rate disappointment and pain in my life (0=high, 10=low) now: _____

24. Overall, I'd rate disappointment and pain in the life of an average person (0=high, 10=low): _____

ASSESSMENT OF HOW LIFE OUGHT TO BECOME AFTER FIBROMYALGIA

Answer on a scale of 0–10 (10 = most, highest, best)

1. Name a job you would most like (and have a reasonable chance of finding) after fibromyalgia: _____

   When healthy, my overall satisfaction with that job ought to be: _____

2. My assessment of how well *I would be able* to perform that job: _____

3. My assessment of how well I expect to *actually* perform that job: _____

4. How satisfying would the salary from this job be? _____

5. My expectations of advancement at this job would be: _____

6. How important will it be for me to fulfill family obligations? _____

7. How do I rate the degree to which I will fulfill family obligations after fibro? _____

8. The amount of pleasure I *would like* from my family: _____

9. The amount of pleasure I *expect* to derive from my family after fibro: _____

10. The degree of pain I *would like* from my family (0=most pain) after fibro: _____

11. The degree of pain I *expect* to derive from my family (0=most pain) after fibro: _____

12. The amount of fun I *expect to have* on my/our next vacation: _____

13. The amount of fun I *expect to actually have* on my/our next vacation: _____

(continued)

ASSESSMENT OF HOW LIFE OUGHT TO BE AFTER FIBROMYALGIA

Answer on a scale of 0–10 (10 = most, highest, best)

C

14. The degree of satisfaction I *would hope to have* on my/our next vacation: _____

15. The degree of satisfaction I *expect to actually have* on my/our last vacation: _____

16. Skip. _____

17. The approximate number of weeks since my/our last vacation: _____

18. The approximate number of days since I last thought about a vacation idea: _____

19. I expect my energy level after fibromyalgia to be: _____

20. Overall, I'd rate the energy level of the average person to be: _____

21. Overall, I expect my satisfaction with my life after fibromyalgia will be: _____

22. Overall, I'd rate the satisfaction of the average person with their life: _____

23. Overall, I expect disappointment and pain in my life after fibromyalgia (0=high, 10=low) will be: _____

24. Overall, I'd rate disappointment and pain in the life of an average person (0=high, 10=low): _____

ASSESSMENT OF LIFE WITH AND WITHOUT FIBROMYALGIA

Transfer your answers from Parts A, B, and C here to columns 2, 3 and 4. Then consult instructions at the bottom of this form.

Assessment of Life with and without Fibromyalgia COLUMN 1	Before Fibromyalgia (Part A) COLUMN 2	Now (Part B) COLUMN 3	After Fibromyalgia (Part C) COLUMN 4	Column 4 minus column 3		Follow-up after being freed from Fibromyalgia COLUMN 6
				COLUMN 5A	COLUMN 5B	
1. Overall job satisfaction						
2. Potential job performance						
3. Actual job performance						
4. Salary satisfaction						
5. Expectations of job advancement						
6. Importance of family obligations						
7. Fulfillment of family obligations						
8. Pleasure *expected* from family						
9. *Actual* pleasure from family						
10. Pain you *expect* from family						

(continued)

ASSESSMENT OF LIFE WITH AND WITHOUT FIBROMYALGIA

Transfer your answers from Parts A, B, and C here to columns 2, 3 and 4. Then consult instructions at the bottom of this form.

Assessment of Life with and without Fibromyalgia COLUMN 1	Before Fibromyalgia (Part A) COLUMN 2	Now (Part B) COLUMN 3	After Fibromyalgia (Part C) COLUMN 4	Column 4 minus column 3		Follow-up after being freed from Fibromyalgia COLUMN 6
				COLUMN 5A	COLUMN 5B	
11. Pain *actually received* from family						
12. Vacation expected fun						
13. Vacation actual fun						
14. Vacation expected satisfaction						
15. Vacation actual satisfaction						
16. Vacation and lovely thoughts						
17. Forward-looking pleasure						
18. Room for fun in life						
19. Energy level						
20. Expected energy level in life						
21. Overall satisfaction with life						

P A R T

D

Assessment of Life with and without Fibromyalgia	Before Fibromyalgia (Part A)	Now (Part B)	After Fibromyalgia (Part C)	Column 4 minus column 3		Follow-up after being freed from Fibromyalgia
COLUMN 1	COLUMN 2	COLUMN 3	COLUMN 4	COLUMN 5A	COLUMN 5B	COLUMN 6
22. Expected satisfaction from life						
23. Overall pain seen in life						
24. Expected pain from life						
25. Example:	5	3	7	+4		
26. Example 2:	6	4	3	–1	+2	

Further things to do with Form 2D: Assessment of Life with and without Fibromyalgia

In all rows except 17 and 18, subtract the figures in column 3 from the figures in column 4. Enter the figures (along with their + or – sign) in column 5A.

In rows 17 and 18, reverse the procedure—subtract the figures in column 4 from the figures in column 3.

Go back to any numbers in column 5A that have a minus sign (–) in front of them. In each such row, subtract the figure in column 3 from the one in column 2. Enter it in column 5B.

Circle any results in columns 5A or 5B that have negative numbers (minus signs).

(continued)

While this is not meant to be a test of your psychological health, we urge you to spend quiet time examining what's going on in those areas in your life where you seem to be getting better results while suffering from fibromyalgia than before you developed it, and better results than you expect to achieve after freedom from fibromyalgia. (That's the general focus of items that end up with at least one negative number after them.) As you start working on the obvious and hidden anger, grief, or shame in your life—in order to keep them from generating the poisons of fibromyalgia—these circled topics should be fruitful areas to delve into as possible causes or effects of your strong emotions. If during any meditation session in the next five weeks you don't know where to start, focus on one of these areas of your life. We believe you will eventually develop the habit of always looking first for underlying emotional causes when you experience any fibromyalgia symptoms. Right now we ask you to practice this as if you are making an emotional inventory.

On a cheerier note, go down column 5A again and locate the five rows with the largest positive numbers. Write a big, bold, happy exclamation mark after those five. Think of them as your high spots. Either your fibromyalgia has robbed you of your pleasure in those things, or the thought of dealing with them after fibro has been exorcised from your life seems mighty pleasant. When you most need to find something positive to hope for in life, these five will be good candidates.

Leave column 6 blank right now. Someday after you've achieved freedom from fibromyalgia, come back and fill it in. Life can be a vacation every day!

I went to a bookstore and asked the sales-
woman, "Where's the self-help section?" She
said if she told me, it would defeat the purpose.
—George Carlin

SIMPLIFY: MAKE ROOM
TO GET BETTER

There's a reason that books with titles like *Simple Abundance* and magazines with titles like *Real Simple* are so popular. People realize that life is overwhelming: too much pain, too many distractions, too many belongings, too many obligations. Many of us want to pare down, to cut back, to eliminate all but the true essentials of life. Most people could use some simplification, but for people with fibromyalgia, it's an absolute necessity. The stress of a hectic life triggers our illness. With our more-sensitive-than-average nervous systems, it makes sense to explore how we can limit sensory input. That alone will lessen our overwhelming sense of system overload.

To help you get rid of some of the chaotic clutter in your life, look first at activities that you can simplify. Become your own efficiency expert.

How do we know you've been living amidst chaos? You've got fibromyalgia, haven't you? If life wasn't chaotic before fibromyalgia, it most certainly is with it. Your sensitive nervous system can turn even the normal bumps in life into overwhelming mountains.

If you've been coping by trying to fight fibromyalgia and maintain a somewhat normal life at the same time, you may have convinced yourself that this chaotic maze of a life is normal. Many sufferers' fundamental problems come from the complications in life that they've learned to take for granted. You may have to step back and take a tough, objective look to identify the mind-sets or roles—yours or other people's—that have become your stumbling blocks. These particular attitudes or interactions may be the main triggers for the repressed anger, grief, or shame that are fueling your fibromyalgia.

To get well, you must unlearn that coping mechanism. It's hard to change everything overnight, but it's easy to simplify your life one aspect at a time, as we'll do during treatment. Give it a try. For each bit of rogue emotion you shake off, you'll also lose some pain!

Simplifying your life might be easier than you think. Betsy told her support group, "The world was going too fast. So I slowed it down—I don't even wear a watch now."

Many people who suffer from fibromyalgia tend to be like Betsy. They've spent their lives shoving relentlessly toward some goal that's always just beyond their reach. If they get close to the goal, they just set the stakes higher. Or they sacrifice their own needs for the sake of someone else's. Both mind-sets boil up lots of anger, a trigger for fibromyalgia symptoms.

You didn't invent these self-defeating outlooks on life, you were taught them. You tend to notice more need around you, and you feel obliged to respond to it. Probably no one ever taught you how to specifically take care of yourself—how to recharge your own batteries. Now we want to teach you how to do it. We want you to be able to say, like Betsy did, "I'm changing, and I like who I'm becoming." When you do, you'll be well on your way to healing. So force yourself out of a self-defeating mind-set by focusing on simplifying your life.

To start, look for and eliminate just one thing that you

o Don't need

o Don't enjoy

o Won't miss

o Think may be dragging you down

Be realistic. Examine your life critically and dispassionately, not as the person living it but from the viewpoint of a hired consultant, a hotshot efficiency expert. Here are some questions you'd do well to ask yourself:

- Do you really need to spend so much time cooking every night? Do you enjoy the effort?

- Do you really need to cook something *every* night? Is it a pleasure? A job? A joke? A bad habit?

- Do the dishes really have to be done before you go to bed, or is that your mother talking to you? Right now, are you the one who's best suited to the job of doing the dishes? Can someone do it for you? You may need others to share the load.

- Would the world fall apart and your family be forced into the poorhouse if you hired someone to clean house once every week or two? House-cleaners are paid to clean around clutter, so don't think you'll have to rush around straightening up in advance. Recognize that kind of thinking as a self-defeating roadblock we perfectionists and goodists create.

- Is it worth saving $20 to drive across town every week and walk for a couple of hours through a football-field-sized supermarket instead of just buying things as you need them at a closer, somewhat more expensive grocery? Can you shop for several weeks' groceries at a time, or order through your computer? (Check out how long milk, eggs, and such keep fresh in modern refrigerators. Beginner cookbooks all have guidelines. Those "sell by" dates aren't "use by" dates!)

Add your own questions here—and answer them with an eye toward simplifying your life. Focus on areas of your life that feel too burdensome, stimulating or overwhelming.

Next, let your consultant (remember, that's you) simplify your life outside the house:

○ Do you really need the money from your job more than an end to fibromyalgia? Do you need it all, or can you cut down your hours or the amount of energy you expend at your job?

○ Which comes first, working on a promotion or working on freedom from fibromyalgia?

○ What would curing fibromyalgia do for your job performance? Shouldn't the curing come first?

○ Do you really get any benefit or pleasure at all right now from your volunteering activities?

○ What kind of supermom or big wheel will you be from a wheelchair, forced there as the fibromyalgia gets worse? (We're not exaggerating to scare you. Every support group we've visited includes some long-term fibromyalgia sufferers in wheelchairs.)

The above list is just a sampling of the kinds of choices we made after consulting with ourselves about our lifestyles. When it comes to your own lifestyle—your own job, family, and priorities—you have to be your own tough, objective consultant who helps find ways to simplify your own life.

Franklynn simplified his life by learning to use the word no comfortably and frequently for the first time in his life. No, he wouldn't volunteer for any new committee no matter how socially vital it was. No, he wouldn't give a speech for any organization no matter how great its goals. No, he wouldn't write a book or article to help out anybody. No, he couldn't take a shift at the homeless men's shelter until his fibromyalgia was gone. And no, he wouldn't even schedule going dancing a couple of weeks in advance, preferring to decide only hours before the event whether he felt up to going. At first he felt slightly guilty saying no to worthwhile causes and people, but as he saw how his fluent use of no helped enormously to simplify his life and crush his fibromyalgia, he delighted in saying no. He still uses the word more now than in his pre-fibromyalgia life. He also got very serious about applying priorities to his work. Instead of sitting at his desk until all of the day's or week's to-do list items were checked off and all e-mail answered, he stacked his lists and e-mail by importance. Must-do items went on top, junk items on the bottom. In between, the hardcore business items always trumped professional courtesies. He slogged through as far as his energies permitted. Leftovers went onto the next day's or next week's piles and were reprioritized with those e-mails and to-dos. Along the way, low-priority tasks fell off the back of his computer monitor and were never seen again—nor missed.

Dr. Selfridge's patient Melissa was accustomed to letting her husband off the hook when it came to house-hold chores. He frequently watched TV in the evening while she finished up the dishes, laundry, and bill-paying after the kids were put to bed. She simplified her life by having him take over bill-paying and consistently doing the dinner dishes so that she could "carve out" some meditation time for herself each day.

Patsy was a gifted baker and would never dream of getting store-bought goodies for any occasion. But she did compromise when she realized that she could use baking time for journaling and meditation.

Nancy decided to teach her kids to cook at a young age and they enjoyed it. So they were already helping substantially with the family meals by the time she started getting free from fibromyalgia. When she needed more time for her treatment program, she started to let the girls make a grocery list and then sent them to the store with a blank check. This took a leap of faith on her part, but they came through with flying colors, though a bag or two extra of chips would sometimes make it home.

Nancy called herself "the original yes woman" until she simplified her life by saying no. She taught her-self to turn down schedule-busting speaking engage-ments, to say no to coffee dates and friends' shopping excursions. She put her newfound extra time into meditation, prayer, and reading—the things that help her recharge and renew. As an extra dividend, her children even felt more tended to.

If you find yourself fumbling for what to simplify first, bring in an outside consultant. Ask a good friend to suggest some possible ways to simplify your life. How about a social worker or other staff person at a medical facility you trust? How about a member of the clergy who knows you and your household well? If you do decide to try the advice of a consultant, line up that person pronto. We're freeing up your time, not wasting it!

Don't take this action, or not take it, to please others. Some of what you simplify may annoy some or all family members to no end. It wouldn't surprise us if you start hearing new complaints as a result of your lifestyle simplification—from your loved ones, people at work, people at your social or religious organizations, friends, or neighbors. You'll need to make believe that you're tough, that you don't care so much how others may judge you. Remember, you're healing. What in the world could be more important?

If you think that there's anything more important than getting well right now, think again. It's nearly impossible to serve two masters, your own health and somebody else's need for the status quo. That conflict may have contributed to your getting fibromyalgia in the first place. It could keep you from recovering now.

If this advice to hang tough sounds cold and uncaring, ask yourself: "Who's in charge here? Who knows best what I need? Who will benefit by my getting well? And who's getting in the way of my treatment?" For everybody who's genuinely concerned with your well-being, the most important thing is your recovery.

When Anna started the program, she saw the importance of simplifying her life, but she couldn't always bring herself to look squarely at her baggage and decide which pieces had to go and which could stay. One day she went to an Al-Anon meeting. She'd gone years earlier with her former spouse, who'd had a drinking problem. Her reason for going this time, she explained, was to hear again "another dose of their philosophy—to change what I can and not sweat the rest. In this course of treatment for fibromyalgia, it's once again been very helpful to me."

Change can be simply relaxing the rules. Betsy describes herself as "a properly raised kind of person"— so well programmed to do the "right" thing that she'd never allowed herself even to write in one of her own books. But as she was reading Dr. Sarno's book, she realized that she'd get more from it if she wrote in her reactions to important ideas. For the first time, she gave herself permission to underline and to make notes on its pages. Betsy says she felt absolutely liberated when she first took pen in hand to write in the book. It's that kind of personal liberation that leads to liberation from fibromyalgia, and it's a good example of the small simplifications with big payoffs we expect you to find and make every day during Weeks Two and Four.

In Chapter Four we told you about Janelle, whose

unsympathetic, uncaring husband had exacerbated her suffering from fibromyalgia for eleven years. One of Janelle's major simplifications was to get him out of her life. For her, it proved to be the most important step on her road toward freedom from fibromyalgia.

Janelle's remedy, though necessary in her case, was extreme. Both of the authors have gone through divorce, and we're not advocating it for any reader of this book. What we want to show here is that some fibromyalgia sufferers may need to face life-altering decisions in order to make their futures manageably healthy. Their goal is to solve deep-seated problems that, like the anger, grief, and shame, have been hiding unacknowledged for a long time.

If you fully acknowledge and accept that chaotic circumstances are triggers for your body symptoms, and if you get chaos out of your life, yet the symptoms don't go away, you may find help in appropriate psychotherapy. We will come back to this point in more detail later.

SIMPLIFY FOREVER

The simplifications that you make can be short-term or long-term changes. You can think of them, if you like, as things to do until you defeat fibromyalgia. You can explain them that way to your family, friends, co-workers, and anybody else. But they're not just to make room for your healing sessions. They're made to get to the roots of your illness. Once you reach freedom from fibromyalgia, you will need to reevaluate your life with respect to those around you. Possibly after consultation with your loved ones and/or family members, you will eventually have to decide which complications will never be compatible with your health. But don't worry about that stage of your recovery now. Apply what energies you still have to changing things day by day.

It's corny but easy to remember, so here goes: A simplification a day keeps the fibromyalgia doctor away!

Self-pity in its early stages is as snug as a
feather mattress. Only when it hardens does it
become uncomfortable.

—Maya Angelou

6 MEDITATE TO ACCESS YOUR MIND

Dr. Selfridge discovered that all her patients who
successfully eliminated their fibromyalgia symptoms had one reflex in common: When physical
symptoms occur, they're able to switch their
focus to the emotions behind the symptoms.
Meditation, a powerful method for quieting
down the mind and increasing self-awareness, is
a valuable tool to help you learn this important
skill of focusing. People who are experienced at
or take quickly to traditional meditation, self-
hypnosis, positive thinking, visualization, or a
similar technique generally overcome their fibromyalgia relatively quickly, since meditation enhances the ability to screen out distractions.

Some patients arrive at Dr. Selfridge's office
with a history of meditating. Others have fre-

quently found comfort listening to motivational tapes, or used similar ways to encourage their brain to work for rather than against them. If you've never meditated before, we'll help you learn to use this practice to heal your fibromyalgia. We'll provide examples of others who've been as sick as you and used it to get well.

We've built in time for meditation sessions in your get-well schedule, beginning in Week Two. They alternate between morning and evening because some people find they work better early in the day, others as the day is drawing to a close. If you find that one time clearly works better for you than the other, switch to that time every day for meditation. If neither time feels significantly better, you can pick the time in which you're least likely to run into potential scheduling conflicts.

A VERY SHORT COURSE IN MEDITATION

People who've never meditated often come to us with misconceptions picked up from skeptics, cartoonists, and their own vivid imaginations. Part of the confusion may be because there are enough meditation styles and techniques to fill an encyclopedia. Since our goal is not to complicate your life but to help you make it simpler, we'll offer a blend of meditation methods that can move you to a place that's fun to be in. It's fun because this is a place where you, and you alone, control the world as you see it at the time. It's a powerful place to battle fibromyalgia—and it's a place where you always win.

If you're already a regular meditator, you should be able to move quickly through this chapter and the next. But please don't skip over them. Instead, compare your methods to ours as you read. You may want to adapt our methods to fit your own style. If you do, pay particular attention to our goals for your meditation sessions.

During meditation, most classic meditators move their minds to a nicer place—or to no place at all. Meditators who have fibromyalgia are no different. They generally whisk themselves away, mentally, to a place that's warm and unconflicted and free of pain. But a dramatically different focus is required if the meditation is going to help root out fibromyalgia.

Before Franklynn met up with Dr. Selfridge, he too used meditation to get to a better place. It did shove his fibromyalgia pains off to one side just far enough so that he could, in a week, crawl through four or five working days and the three vigorous aerobic workouts prescribed by his general practitioner.

For the workouts, he'd get to the gym early enough to claim a secure corner spot and meditate himself far away to a small, sunny island with a waterfall. He'd watch himself as a young boy with his grandmother, doing not much of anything except feeling good, warm, and secure, all the while doing the "grasshoppers" and "pop turns" and other choreographed aerobic movements without leaving his meditative state. Usually people gave him room to stay in his dream state. They noticed that he never seemed totally aware of what was going on around him.

Then Dr. Selfridge introduced Franklynn to the body chemistry that was fueling his fibromyalgia. She explained that his repressed anger was provoking fibromyalgia-making chemicals, and that he'd have fibromyalgia for as long as he failed to recognize that his emotions were the source of his symptoms. She also explained how he could use meditation to help him look intently inward toward these emotions.

So Franklynn stopped meditating to distract himself from his pain and, instead, focused through it to whatever kind of anger he could find rumbling around in his life. He found more wells of it than he believed possible, and within a few weeks this recognition turned off his fibromyalgia pain.

Be sure to schedule your meditation. On the printed schedule, we've started you off with thirty minutes a day, shortening the time to twenty to twenty-five minutes after you get the hang of it. If you're an old hand at meditating, you may be able to start with twenty-minute sessions and possibly cut down to fifteen minutes by our final week. But when in doubt, schedule more time rather than less.

CREATE THE BEST MEDITATION ATMOSPHERE

Silence is golden when you're a new meditator. If you have a room or some other space where you can count on no interruptions, noises, or other distractions, that's the place to go. If you don't, here's a kit to help you turn almost any room into a workable meditation environment.

Put a sign on the door: Recovering from Fibromyalgia. Please Do Not Disturb. If there are children or others in the house who can't read or won't always obey signs, you'll need to explain what this sign means and warn them that once you're in the room you'll ignore all knocks on the door (though not warnings like "Fire!").

Locate some classical or easy-listening music, without words, that is so familiar it won't sneak up and capture your attention. Pick something soothing, to help you generate as many "up" chemicals as possible. Position the music player where it will block out any outside noise. Adjust the volume so that it's just loud enough to mask extraneous noises but not so loud as to take over your attention.

If pressure or worry makes you have to go to the bathroom, go now.

Find a chair that supports your back and will feel comfortable for a full half hour.

Set an alarm clock for thirty minutes, but if it ticks, put it near the music source so you don't hear the ticking. Turn the clock so you can't see the time. Take off your watch and put it out of reach.

Lock the door if it has a lock. (If it doesn't, you may want to install one.)

Sit down. Here we go.

TEACH YOURSELF TO RELAX

Meditation is a very old, very safe, and effective way to focus your energies on what's important. What is important? We'll assume that what's important for you is to heal your fibromyalgia. After that, you might like to use the control that meditation gives you over your life and your priorities to help you decide what else is important. Meditating can make good things happen and make bad things go away. Many recovered fibromyalgia patients continue using it to help them fine-tune their lives.

In meditation, we want to channel all possible physical energy into the mind. One of the best ways to make physical energy available to our mental faculties is to relax as completely as possible.

You may be worrying that your fibromyalgia will get in the way of relaxing. You may have forgotten how to relax. You may fear you'll be distracted by the pain. Remember, we are not practicing meditation to escape or smother that pain, as Franklynn used to do. It can be done, but the results don't last long. We meditate to focus on the anger (or shame or grief) that's making the biochemicals that are causing fibromyalgia. Your body's pain is a way that your mind distracts you from facing up to the painful emotions lurking there.

So if pain is a constant part of your life, let it alone. Follow the progression of relaxation exercises that we present here, and for now let the pain coexist with your relaxed self.

Start by sitting comfortably. Don't twist yourself into any unusual positions. Just sit normally in a comfortable chair. (Later—after you've mastered meditation—if you want to try another position, do it.) Rest your feet on the floor, with your posture erect. Be sure your arms and hands will remain comfortable in the position they're now in for the next half hour. Think about lifting the top of your head as close to heaven as possible. Good posture helps you sit longer in one position without becoming distracted by parts of your body.

Relax your body parts one by one, starting at the top and working down. Here's how:

Close your eyes gently. Focus on your forehead. Let go of whatever tension you find there. Let the frowns and wrinkles flatten out. You may feel a tiny amount of upward pull on your eyebrows. Feel the pleasure of that pull.

Relax your ears.

Let your jaw hang loose. If your mouth opens, that's okay. You're alone.

Now focus your mind on your entire head. Relax the whole head as one unit. During this step, you may find that some part of your head is not yet relaxed enough. Focus on it again and make it relax. Then go back to thinking of your entire head as one unit, and deliberately but gently relax the whole wonderful head.

Relax your neck. It connects your head to your strong body. If it helps, move your neck slightly at first so you can get feedback about how relaxed it really is.

(Eventually you'll remain nearly motionless during meditation.)

Most of us start out with tons of tension concentrated in our shoulders. Relax them—first the right one and then the left. Don't forget your shoulder blades. After they're both relaxed, inspect your head, neck, and shoulders as a unit. Be sure you haven't tensed up any part of them as you concentrated on relaxing something else.

Relax your arms, first the right one and then the left.

Relax your hands, first the right and then the left. You may get the best results by focusing on each finger, one by one, until each hand stops feeling like a separate part of your body.

We'll get to your spine and torso in a minute, when we focus on breathing.

Relax your legs and feet, first the right, then the left. Start at the hip, then move to the knee. You may want to adjust the relative position of your legs so they'll feel more relaxed. If you do, remember to start meditating with your legs in this position tomorrow. Mentally reach down to the ankle and relax it. Then toe by toe, starting at the smallest toe, searching for tension and insisting on relaxation. Now move on to the other leg, relaxing from hip to toes.

Don't worry about how long this relaxation process takes. With practice, you'll move quickly into a state of total comfort and relaxation. The completeness of your relaxation is more important than your speed.

BREATHE TO RELAX

Breathing is the next key element in meditation. Breathe in through your nose and breathe out through your mouth. Breathing out through your mouth helps keep your jaw loose and your teeth unclenched despite tension or fibromyalgia pain. If you have nasal or sinus congestion or a similar problem and you find that this pattern interferes with relaxation, let the air go both ways through your mouth or through your nose.

Focus all of your attention now on your breathing. Breathe deeper. As you inhale, fill your lungs completely but not uncomfortably. Empty your lungs completely as you exhale.

With your eyes still closed, visualize your breathing. Watch your lungs expand to take in fresh, clean air. Watch them squeeze out the used-up, stale air.

After a while, with your eyes still closed, visualize the air expanding throughout your whole body, renewing it with fresh oxygen. Then watch as your body expels all the old air with its pain.

Deliberately observe the rate of your breathing. If it slows down or speeds up, ask yourself why. Are you nervous? Overeager? Acknowledge these sensations, but don't judge them. Let them go and return to steady breaths. Once you're confident moving through these steps into profound meditation and you've experienced the pleasures it can bring you, you may automatically slow down the number of breaths you take. If you feel you're breathing too fast, consciously intervene to slow things down a bit. But always make adjustments gradually. Don't insist on perfection or try so hard to follow our instructions that you risk getting panicky or uncomfortable. If that happens, just start this meditation exercise all over again.

FOCUS ON FOCUSING

Fibromyalgia sufferers typically spend much of their time focusing on pain, moving from "What is this new pain?" to "Will it get worse?" to "What should I take for it?" to "Should I change my plans?" The relaxation you've just achieved has helped you, however briefly, to forget about your body. That brief moment is long enough to start teaching your body and brain to turn off fibromyalgia.

With fibromyalgia, it's your body that hurts, but the production of the chemicals responsible for those pains is triggered in a part of the mind that most people don't communicate with very often. When we fully relax the body, the mind moves into position to turn off those nasty chemicals. It can put a halt to the negative cascade of thoughts that accompanies each onset of pain.

During ordinary undirected meditation, the point is to keep the mind unfocused. In some classic meditation styles, chanting a Buddhist mantra (such as om) over and over is a way to unfocus. In other techniques, you actually focus on unfocusing. These methods are valuable for setting your mental energies in a general path, such as preparing to do your best thinking during a workday.

But for our purposes, we can't let the mind go its own way. If we do that, it will take us deep into the swamp called fibromyalgia. Besides, here and now we have a specific goal in mind: to redirect the mind from doing what it normally does for us, because right now that includes getting the brain to generate fibromyalgia-fueling biochemicals. We need to refocus it in a way that tricks the brain and turns off those biochemicals. Our program calls for a directed meditative state, one in which you substitute thoughts that thwart your brain's strategy of creating fibromyalgia symptoms to distract you from your conscious emotions.

We start by savoring the magnificent feeling that comes from focusing all our energies onto one small doable task. So imagine a place that's very nice to look at—inside a majestic building, perhaps, or somewhere in the great outdoors. Since you don't have to pay for it, let your imagination soar. Really give in to your whims. Give that place a waterfall, ocean, rainbow, sumptuous view, or museum-quality art collection—whatever you most want in your space. Make the climate just right for you, whether warm, windy, or cool. Adjust the sounds in this virtual space to please your taste right now. Classical music, jazz, angels on golden harps, meadow-larks—your imagination's the limit. One other thing to remember: no talking allowed, not even virtually. If there's somebody, real or not, who can make your private place warm and fuzzy for you, put them there in your meditative mind. But don't let either of you speak.

Go there, be there, enjoy it. If it's not a wonderful place to be for you right now, then redesign it. You ought to feel good going there and being there, really good. Stay there until your thirty-minute alarm brings you back to your real room.

As you're relaxing and breathing slowly and deeply, your mind may drift off or focus on something that seems unrelated to what we're doing right now. That's normal. Don't worry about it. If it happens, notice where your mind drifted to: a place, a person, an event, something on your mind? There may be significance to the where, who, or what. Then again, there may be none at all.

If your mind drifts to the same place several times, we can assume there's something going on there that you ought to think about seriously. But this is probably not the best time for you to do that thinking. When meditating, we strive to reach a different relationship with our minds than when we're actively thinking about some particular subject. So once you've noted where your mind has taken you, focus again on your breathing to make it go back to your wonderful place.

When you focus all of your body energy and mental powers on this one job, it's like holding a magnifying glass so that it catches the sun. That lens condenses the sun's energies into a tiny spot, and that spot soon becomes hot enough to set fire to paper or wood.

Nobody gets to Camelot on the first try. Success is catching a glimpse, however small, of the peace you feel when you really do focus a major share of your mental energies on a single goal and when you look forward to getting there again and again. It doesn't take any special skills, just patience and practice.

Soon we'll work together to harness this powerful peace of mind to unseat fibromyalgia. We won't go in search of a pleasant place to hide from it. Instead, we'll find and disarm the hidden emotion generating the biochemicals that put us in fibromyalgia's grip. You'll know you're ready for this next step (Chapters 7 and 8) when you can move quickly through all the preliminary steps of relaxing and arriving in your favorite scene. Eventually you may find a favorite personal image that triggers the meditation state. You've already heard about Franklynn's warm, sunny island. With it in mind, he speeds through his mental checklist, relaxing, breathing, and quickly getting to a virtual space where he feels warm, pain-free, and secure.

When Frances, a facilitator for a metropolitan hospital's fibromyalgia support group, wants to meditate, she imagines a deep well. By the time she drops her red pail on a rope deep into the cold, clear water, she's totally focused and ready for the next step.

If after four or five sessions you still don't feel the tranquillity we've described, stop and reread this chapter.

If you still aren't sure you're getting its pain-relieving benefits, read more about meditation or enroll in a session with a meditation teacher. In the Resources section, we describe books and other resources that can help support your recovery. Almost every community now has experienced instructors; some are on hospital and clinic staffs. Don't worry about which "brand" of meditation to pick. Instead, pick the facilitator you feel most comfortable with. Show the person this chapter and Chapter 7 to help him or her understand your reasons for wanting to meditate. If the individual is willing to help, you'll have a powerful ally.

Meditation is a major tool in conquering fibromyalgia. You're also likely to find it rewarding throughout the rest of your pain-free life.

Many are stubborn in pursuit of the path they
have chosen, few in pursuit of the goal.
—Friedrich Nietzsche

CUT OLD ANGERS
DOWN TO SIZE

Once you've become relatively comfortable with
meditating to relax and feel good for the moment,
you're ready to refocus your meditative energies
in a way that helps free you in the long term
from fibromyalgia pain. We are now going to
help focus your energies on unconscious anger,
the anger that you've hidden underneath layers
of defenses. You are human, and part of being
human is having some kind of hidden anger,
shame, or grief. You might identify it more
easily by some of its aliases—fury, frustration,
repressed anger, rage. You might experience it as
sadness, boredom, lack of motivation, low self-
esteem, or just not ever feeling well.

Perhaps you believe you don't have any
anger, hidden or otherwise. Dr. Selfridge saw

herself for many years as "nice Nancy," never acknowledging any of those "uncivilized" feelings. We regularly visit fibromyalgia support groups on the Internet where the vocal majority denies having anger of any kind. Then those same people type in long, sad treatises about their pained and drained bodies. We find it very frustrating; if those people would only put that much feeling into rooting out their unacknowledged anger, they're likely to heal.

For patients who find it hard to accept that they too hide the normal, human unconscious rage and similar intense emotions that fuel fibromyalgia, Dr. Selfridge uses the example of how the military trains soldiers. All over the world, she points out, governments are able to attract into military service many young, healthy people with normal psychological profiles, from normal, functional families. In short, they start out like the rest of us. Then, in the basic training designed to prepare them for combat, higher-ranking, experienced individuals challenge the recruits' independence by curbing their freedom and pouring on offensive demoralizations. Within several weeks, the recruits have been taught to tap into enough fear and rage that they can kill with their bare hands. The ease with which reprogramming takes place is enough to turn the stomach of anyone not similarly trained, and it works only because it reaches down into the anger that is inside all of us, basic to our human fiber, part of our evolutionary baggage. Rage is not psychopathology, and it is not our "fault."

You can embrace the fact that you are human and have subconscious anger, and be rid of your fibromyalgia. Or you can fight over whether or not you even have anger hidden somewhere in your tired head or aching muscles, in which case you're likely to live with fibromyalgia a long time. The wiser course is to accept that subconscious anger is there in your sensitive nervous system.

To show how many events in our lives have a real, demonstrable impact on triggering the rage that gives us fibromyalgia, we'll update the list of stressors published in Dr. Sarno's *The Mindbody Prescription*, which was developed by two pioneering New York physicians, Dr. Thomas Holmes and Dr. Richard Rahe, after studying the effects of stressful living on what they called "the natural history of many diseases." The list is organized so the events most likely to trigger fibromyalgia are at the top of the list. While many of these events trigger unresolved grief and shame, buried anger—the primitive "why me" emotion—is the longest-lingering component and often the hardest to acknowledge.

○ Death of a spouse

○ Divorce

○ Marital separation

○ Jail term

○ Death of a close family member

○ Personal injury or illness

- Marriage

- Loss of job

- Marital reconciliation

- Retirement

- Change in health of a family member

- Pregnancy

- Sex difficulties

- Addition of a new family member

- Business readjustment

- Change in financial condition

- Death of a close friend

- Change to a different line of work

- Change in number of arguments with spouse

- Mortgage over $20,000

- Foreclosure of mortgage or loan

- Change of responsibilities at work

- Son or daughter leaving home

- Trouble with in-laws

- Outstanding personal achievement

- Spouse begins or stops work

- Begin or end school

- Change in living conditions

- Revision of personal habits

- Trouble with boss

- Change in work hours or conditions

- Change in residence

- Change in schools

- Change in recreation

- Change in religious activities

- Change in social activities

- Mortgage or loan of less than $20,000

- Change in sleeping habits

- Change in number of family get-togethers

- Change in eating habits

- Vacation

- Christmas

- Minor violation of the law[46]

Please note that some of these life events are presumably situations you'd welcome, such as a reconciliation, vacation, or major holiday. However, they can still cause stress and tension, revving up a cycle of self-doubt or anger. You can love Christmas but still feel stressed out by its demands. You can welcome a new job but still have to cope with the tumultuous emotions of leaving your old job and worrying about what's ahead.

REACH FOR THE ANGER

Remember back a few chapters where we detailed the physical, biochemical, and emotional underpinnings of this complex illness we call fibromyalgia? We didn't say you got fibromyalgia because you get angry. Appropriately expressed anger is good, not bad. Most of its physical effects are well understood: Your heart rate goes up, your blood pressure goes up, and you secrete increased levels of stress hormones such as adrenaline and noradrenaline.

But if you're like most of us, you probably feel some kind of guilt or shame about having anger. "Good" people swallow it. Some of us with fibromyalgia were brought up feeling that way. Some wouldn't dream of humiliating ourselves by openly showing rage. Some, because of our heightened sensitivity, suppress it to avoid conflict. But these suppressed emotions are the ones that can eventually lead to fibromyalgia.

Frankly, nobody can say for certain why, in some people, their pain peptides "go wild." Nobody knows yet what kinds of medications or inoculations—if any—will be able to control it in the future. We do know that the symptoms—the pain, the tiredness, the nervous legs, and such—can usually be overcome in patients who let us show them how to accept the emotional source of their symptoms and systematically focus on their emotions rather than their physical signs. That's a treatment we can start today.

Now's the time to do something constructive about it. Give yourself permission to accept that any anger or accompanying guilt is okay, even if you prefer not to openly express it.

If you're still doubtful about having hidden anger, you're unlikely to have experienced any guilt about it so far. Expect it, though, and accept it as a normal part of your healing process. It too will go away.

As a very young infant, you got angry plenty of times. And you expressed it, generally at the top of your lungs. It's a natural thing to do. Sometimes your anger got you fed, changed, or picked up. More often it probably got you nothing but a sore throat. But you still kept getting angry.

As a child, you got angry plenty of times. You expressed it with temper tantrums. It's a natural thing to do. At that age, it's likely your anger consistently got you nothing that felt good, and the lack of result had a strong impact on you, given your sensitive nature. But it couldn't stop you from getting angry.

You no doubt still got angry, on occasion, after you reached adulthood. It's a natural thing to do. But society forbids us to act on our anger, natural or not. You can't hit your kids or your spouse without risking repercussions. You'd better not yell at your boss, your creditors, or even a telephone solicitor. Fearing anger's power over you and the consequences of acting out if you lose control, you avoid the whole mess by denying anger from its very inception.

The very people who seem to walk through life calm, never frazzled, never threatened, are most likely the "goodists" or perfectionists who've learned to internalize and deny their anger. These apparent copers, who seem to let horrible situations roll off their backs, may in fact be squirreling away bushels of rage.

But we're all rugged individualists. Each of us buries our anger in different ways. To help you deal with your own anger, we'll start by seeking the very specific, very individual way in which you hide it away. Remember, we're on a search for the sources of your unconscious rage—and the very search for it can heal you even when you don't consciously find the source.

FIND SPECIFIC ANGER

You can't, as a rule, effectively attack anger in general. You have to focus on individual instances, on specific feelings, individuals, times, and places. Anger happens one incident at a time, so you have to take inventory one incident at a time if you hope to force fibromyalgia out of your life. Complicating the matter further, you don't always see anger when it happens, and the anger that hides is often the most damaging. So you may have to find emotions you never consciously knew were there.

The interesting thing about the subconscious mind is that many, if not all, emotional memories from the past are stored there and can stir up our neuropeptides if properly provoked. This is why an examination of childhood wounds is so important to analytical therapists. Though we want you to try to dig and find any old sources of rage in your life that might be fueling your current symptoms, we know that this is difficult, even with the guidance of a skilled therapist. Fortunately, the "digging" is more important than the "finding." We know that your brain will recognize that you are redirecting your energies toward your emotions, that you are not being distracted by the physical pain that it is creating for you, and eventually the pain will subside— even if you do not find any "issues" that are particularly dramatic.

Look at all the important, contentious, or difficult parts of your life. Go at it like an Anger Cop. Be especially alert for things that you know, rationally, ought to make you angry but don't seem to. Those are likely to be major sources of the repressed anger that fuels your fibromyalgia. Do you rationalize your teenager's rudeness? Did your boss just dump an extra load on your desk, which you accepted without complaint? When your friend stood you up, did you tell her it was not a big deal? Ask yourself: why didn't you get angry?

We don't want you to go around angry. But do become aware of anything that makes you clench your fists, grit your teeth, bite your tongue. When something anger-provoking comes to mind, don't "forget" it or add it to a mental list of things you'll take care of later; if you do, you'll be feeding your fibromyalgia fire. Instead, it's important to write it down on an Anger List that you will review repeatedly during your treatment. Carry a small pad or palm-sized computer everywhere you go. Label the list My Fibro Anger List and give it a date. Below we'll show you how we structured our list.

As you add to your list, don't leave out small angers. Include everything that makes you angry now, that ever made you angry before, everybody and every situation that now stirs you to anger or who ever stirred up your anger. Nothing is too insignificant for this list, nothing too foolish, nothing too long ago to matter anymore, nothing too sacred to touch. This will be between you and your muse, so nobody else will ever know what you write down on your Anger List. But you will know, and it will help you.

Don't expect to be able to completely fill in the last two columns now, when you dredge up the anger. In later treatment sessions, meditation and other techniques will help you find their real source and put them to rest.

Here's a glance at parts of one of Franklynn's Anger Lists:

Summarize the anger	Locate it in time	Identify the source	Describe how you got rid of it
Late to health club	Monday P.M.	Judi	Faced up to the fact that I got warmed up okay anyway, and usually do
A key vendor didn't return essential questionnaire in time for newsletter deadline	Wednesday A.M.	Deleted for privacy	Wrote candidly about vendor's sloppiness in comparison chart's comments section
Phone slammer made a pest of herself during a TV Mozart opera	Thursday evening	Deleted for privacy	Yelled at telemarketer and threatened FTC and FCC action

Here's a glance at selections from one of Nancy's Anger Lists:

Summarize the anger	Locate it in time	Identify the source	Describe how you got rid of it
Another formulary change from the HMO	Monday A.M.	Pharmacy and Therapeutics Committee	Complained (again) to office colleagues, clinic manager, finally the chairman of the committee about how much more work this generates for me as patients call to get their long-standing prescriptions changed to the new drugs

Summarize the anger	Locate it in time	Identify the source	Describe how you got rid of it
Kids left six pairs of shoes in the doorway—again.	Wednesday P.M.	Leah, Rachel	Hid shoes in the back of the closet so they'll be "missing" when they need them
Favorite eye-liner pencil missing again when I'm trying to get ready for work	Friday 5 A.M.!	Leah or Rachel	Woke them both up early to extract a confession and teach a lesson to put back the things that they "borrow"

ALWAYS FORGET TODAY'S ANGER TODAY

We want you to learn more about anger than just how to meditate on it. We want you to get a life, not put yourself through daily treatment sessions simply to cope. If that's what it takes, it's better than suffering with fibromyalgia, but you can learn to deal with anger, before it becomes rage, before it turns around and attacks you as fibromyalgia.

Rage itself does not directly hurt our bodies, disrupt our sleep, or sap our energy. What rage does is to force explosions of neuropeptides that cause the specific bodily changes involved in physical pain, sleep disturbances, and fatigue. If you can stop the first explosions from happening—cut the link between the mind's anger and the effects on the body—you can be free from fibromyalgia.

Anna shared with us how she applied what she's learned about anger the day her dentist insulted her. She buried the emotion, as usual, but soon noticed she was hurting physically. Later that day she made the connection between the event and her new pain. She talked to her husband about it. That started the healing process. Then she talked to the dentist's hygienist, who listened attentively and sympathetically. That completed her acknowledgment of the anger. It went away, and the pain left with it. Notice that she never had to directly confront the insulting dentist. Giving vent to her anger was sufficient. (She also dumped the dentist, but that's another book.)

What's the absolute number one best way to avoid storing up anger? Get angry! Get assertive! Interact! If somebody does something to you that you think they shouldn't have done, it's a perfectly normal, healthy, wonderful thing to get angry. It's what humans do. It's how sharing and caring people in society let each other know, "Hey, you've done something that made me very upset. You probably should not have done that, but maybe you're not even aware of what you did." We know that's easier said than done, but time spent rethinking anger can help us understand that getting angry with someone is more intimate and caring than walking away quietly but mad as hell. Healing fibromyalgia depends not on turning into an aggressive person, but on accepting the anger within and at least acknowledging it now and again. You don't need to be a jerk to be assertive when expressing your anger.

Notice how we phrased the above: "You *probably* should not have done that." Maybe you think it shouldn't have happened. Maybe whoever you're angry at thinks it should have. Either way, the problem is real. So stomp your feet and forget it, or think about it straightforwardly, or talk about it and forgive, and then have done with it. But don't bury it down where it can release those ugly messenger chemicals that give you fibromyalgia.

Are you afraid of your anger? Do you think you can slip out of control? If the way you treat other people when you're angry frequently gets you in hot water—at work, bowling, playing bridge, at family functions, wherever—then maybe you need to learn how to get angry in a more socially acceptable way. There are books and community organizations that teach people just that. In the Resources section, we've listed a way to find one. We found one technique in an unexpected place— the novel *Tales of Burning Love*, by Louise Erdrich. In it, a psychology professor explains to the rough-cut hero how to live with his anger: "She told Jackie to mentally image a wire cage, to visualize himself putting up the chain-link, and then to get right inside the damn thing like an animal. She told him that he could pace inside the cage, he could go wild, he could let off his steam as though he had just been captured in the jungle. The only thing was, he had to stay in the cage, not jump the fence, not ever let himself out until he knew he was good and ready."[47] If you think you're getting out of control, imagine your own cage, get inside, and let off steam in the safety of that space. It'll help you like it helped Jackie.

CALL IT ANGER AND GET ON WITH IT

Life will be more fun when you don't have to focus on anger, whether it's past, present, future, potential, or repressed. And that will happen. Once you've completed the exercises in this book, you'll have a clean slate. Anger will come and go. You'll notice it, perhaps jot it down, and then, in effect, erase it. At the slightest recurrence of a fibromyalgia symptom, you'll know to look for—and squelch—the anger that's fueling it. No other thoughts about your symptoms will be entertained.

Do keep updating your Anger List for about a year. After that, you may want to replace it with a mental list. From time to time, stop and carefully check in with your body. If you're effectively keeping the pain out of your life, it's proof positive that your mental list is working for you. If not, go back to writing it down.

A ONE-MINUTE ANGER MANAGER

If you're lucky enough, your special fibro spot may signal when you've got new anger that needs to be dealt with. As we mentioned, Franklynn's left biceps starts aching when he's not effectively processing new anger. As soon as he acknowledges it—a quick 1-2-3 for him now—the biceps quits aching and he's confident that the anger won't cook up fibromyalgia. Cynthia's knees start to ache when she ignores anger, reminding her to face it then and there. Whether or not you have a consistent "fibro spot"—Nancy and many of her patients don't—practice the following One-Minute Anger Manager until it becomes instinctive. Use it the instant you feel pain of any kind anywhere, or as soon as you detect any of the telltale anger reactions: clenched fists, toes, or teeth; held breath. Ask yourself—and answer—these six questions:

○ Who caused the anger?

○ What caused the anger?

○ Why was what they did aimed at me?

○ When did the anger really start?

○ Where will it lead?

○ How should I deal with it?

Remember, it is not necessary to identify and resolve angers with any amount of detail. It isn't even necessary to confront the person who's the source of your anger directly. It is very necessary that you internally identify each and every source of new anger that might contribute to your fibromyalgia, and also figure out who triggered the anger and all of the other details in the above list. The process of confronting anger on your own is generally sufficient to keep it from becoming repressed and then turning into fibromyalgia. Here are some proven ways to accomplish this that we use and that patients report are much easier to use than they at first thought they'd be.

MORE WAYS TO DEFUSE ANGER OVER THE LONG TERM

When Dr. Selfridge first learned about the mind-body technique, she found herself intimidated by the idea of having to dredge up her anger. A conflict avoider from childhood, during her divorce she'd buried intense anger and grief. Her first reaction now was, "If I have to relive *that*, forget it! I'll keep my symptoms!" She discovered that many patients felt the same way.

But there are ways to approach angry thoughts and situations with little likelihood that they will blow up on you. There are useful skills that will help you manage any fears of angry conflict you may have. They can help you attack anger as you meet it, but in ways that don't generate more of that awful stuff.

CHANGE THE WAY YOU THINK WHEN YOU'RE ANGRY

Instead of telling yourself, "It's the most awful thing ever," "It's humiliating," or "I get all the blame," use less damaging expressions like "It's frustrating," "It's silly," or "Getting angry will only make it worse." We are sensitive enough as is, and catastrophic thoughts can't possibly lead to good brain biochemistry for us.

CHOOSE YOUR WORDS CAREFULLY

Teach yourself a new set of words to use when you're facing angry confrontations with others. Get rid of *always* and *never*. Avoid cursing. Whether talking to yourself or to others, try to express anger without forcing the other person or yourself into a corner. Talk only about the specific incident; don't dredge up past or related events.

Try a time-honored technique called the "I" message. For example: "I get angry when you leave your shoes in front of the door after I have told you that I want you to put them away because I feel like you are not listening to me and that you disrespect me. I would like you to show your respect for me by putting away your shoes every time."

What if the situation is a bad one and calls for really tough measures? Put it off. Later, by yourself, defuse it through meditation or journaling (we'll explain the technique of keeping a journal in Chapter 8). Count on these ways to dump the anger without dumping your relationship with whoever is involved. These strategies will help you feel less fearful about facing your anger toward others.

Often when a confrontation is at risk of getting too hot to handle, then taking a time-out is a good idea. It is okay to call the time-out and resume the "discussion" when heads are cooler and problems can be articulated and solved more rationally. Nancy often resorts to nonverbal grunts, nods, and um-hums when her teenagers start an angry barrage. They get to vent and it doesn't turn into WWIII.

COMMUNICATE MORE EFFECTIVELY

Anger makes you speak faster, say a lot more, and listen less. It's a dangerous combination. Many hostile situations are the result of misspoken or misheard words.

Especially when you're angry, make it a point of speaking slowly and deliberately. Remember to choose your words carefully. Listen intently. That's so important that motivational author Stephen Covey makes it one of the seven habits of highly successful people: "Seek first to understand, then to be understood."[48]

ENGAGE IN PROBLEM SOLVING

If you see a way out of an anger-provoking situation, suggest it. It may not be obvious to others. Make the suggestion out loud—in carefully chosen, carefully spoken words. A solution's more likely to work if everyone's in on it.

Be prepared to consider other suggestions. Yours may not be the best. If none is offered and tensions continue, ask if there's a potential solution that you haven't seen or heard about.

You can also attack problems this way if anger wells up when you're alone. For example, if your commute to work frequently triggers anger, change your route or mode of transportation. Once you identify the problem, give yourself a deadline for coming up with a solution. Then try it out.

FIX WHAT YOU CAN SO IT DOESN'T TRIGGER ANGER

Some places trigger anger by association. If you get angry seeing toys strewn around a child's room as you walk by, perhaps because of all the times you tried to teach the child not to leave a messy room, don't look. Or tell the child to keep the door closed. This is one time you ought to take the path of least resistance.

CHANGE YOUR PATTERNS

Most of us fall into certain behavioral patterns, doing a certain thing in a certain way at a certain time. When what we habitually do produces negative emotion, anger can become habitual—a response to the slightest reminder of the anger-provoking situation. The way to deal with this is to break the chain of associations. So if you and your spouse tend to get into fights at bedtime, quit discussing controversial issues at bedtime. Save them for weekends, or try a phone call during lunch. Be creative! It might be necessary, at first, to avoid discussing anything at all at bedtime. If your partner is intent on a late-night "dump" session, keep your distance. Watch TV, read, or play Scrabble or solitaire instead. Make it clear that you're not mad at your partner, that you're not avoiding anything but the habitual angry words that often accompany bedtime.[49]

Notice that these anger-managing routines aren't intended to analyze the particulars and judge who's the good guy and who's the bad guy. We're not counseling you on your marriage or your job, or trying to tell you how to make wonderful friends and have a happy family. We just hope you'll boldly admit to and reflect on the anger before it creates bigger problems for you. This is self-defense against fibromyalgia.

MEDITATING ON ANGER

Much of the meditation you'll do in this program will invite you to focus on a specific instance of anger. Sometimes when you attack effectively and forcefully the anger that's trapped inside, you lose track of other things going on around you. This "crib sheet" can help you quickly and effectively move your mind back to a focused meditative condition each time you're ready to attack new anger.

* * *

Make the room quiet and comfortable

Relax

> Head

> Neck

> Shoulders

> Arms, hands, fingers

> Legs, feet, toes

Breathe deliberately, slowly

Focus

Focus on something wonderful

Focus on anger and eliminate it

* * *

We are confronted with insurmountable opportunities.

—Pogo

CHAPTER 8

JOURNALING, SELF-TALK, AND VISUALIZATION

While directed meditation, which we introduced in Chapter 6, is the most powerful tool for healing fibromyalgia, keeping a journal also helps you open the path to your deepest emotions. Used in tandem, the two techniques make a formidable anti-fibromyalgia kit. Keeping a journal is easy and inexpensive. Many people find it the most satisfying of all the fibromyalgia-healing techniques. Others enjoy self-talk or visualization best; they too can project you into a healthy future.

First let's help you focus your journaling in a way particularly suited to fighting fibromyalgia. It's similar to maintaining a diary. But there are important differences between recording an event or a few insights at day's end and a deliberate effort to root out fibromyalgia by writing in a journal. Most store-bought diaries limit the amount of space available for writing during any one day, but in journaling we encourage you to be as expansive as you care to be.

In order for journaling to be effective against fibromyalgia, we're going to lay down some rules that will help focus it at the right targets. Most important: Do not write about your pains and other symptoms. It's counterproductive, so we absolutely forbid it. Don't write about the temperature, what activities you've done (or left undone), what you ate, how well or poorly you slept, or what medicine you took. They all have little to do with what causes your fibromyalgia and what you can do to get rid of it. Consider all those thoughts your brain's way of distracting you from confronting the anger, grief, or shame that may be boiling up inside you. That's what you must focus on now.

Here is the absolute bottom line: You must think about an experience that provoked enough anger that you couldn't stand to see it, feel it, or remember it. Fortunately, it is absolutely not necessary to relive or even to amicably resolve that experience in order to purge the effects of the hidden anger and its resulting witches' brew of damaging biochemicals.

Recall our earlier discussion of where fibromyalgia comes from: those strong emotions you've stored, hidden, repressed, or avoided. (Reread Chapters 3 or 7 if you need to refresh your memory.) Most people initially have some problems admitting to and facing down these hidden feelings. If it were simple, you wouldn't have hidden them in the first place. Like meditation, journaling is a way to get to a mental place where you can confront the repressed emotions that are crippling your muscles and overwhelming your brain.

Let's consider what it means to confront these feelings, and how you can do it in your journal. You don't have to confront the actual people, places, or things. You don't have to face the feelings themselves to dissipate their power. You do have to hunt hard to find them so you can acknowledge that they exist. It is essential to realize that unconscious emotions remain unconscious unless you work to reveal them. Journaling allows you to simply meet the repressed emotions at the doorway to the unconscious—to just stand there knowing they are there behind the door, causing physical problems. This process seems sufficient to stop the chemical cascade that produces your symptoms. That's why you must spend time thinking about their possible emotional triggers, even if no dramatic emotions ever come to your conscious awareness.

If you locate a source of anger, you don't have to find your way back to its underlying cause. Don't try to resolve it with the person who initiated the anger, whether it was your boss today or your partner this week or a parent twenty or more years ago. Trying to resolve an old situation may diminish the anger, but just as often it could add new anger. Jennifer finally stopped trying to explain to her eighty-year-old father why she still had a grudge about his refusal to support her wish to go to college; she finally realized that he'd considered college a waste of time for women. Instead, she started tracking down in her journal the unacknowledged rage at all of her father's put-downs during her early years.

Often the hardest part of this exercise is continuing to chase down a buried crippling emotion when there's no conscious feedback that you're getting anywhere. But doing this on a regular basis ultimately, and often quickly and thoroughly, eradicates symptoms.

CREATING A JOURNAL

The best format for your special journaling is a bound book of lined paper. If you get a choice of narrow-ruled or wide-ruled paper, choose the wide-ruled, or double-space your writing—later you may want to write some afterthoughts between the lines. Steer clear of journals already formatted with topical headings or dated pages unless you know you'll be able to ignore them entirely.

A diary with a lock and key is useful, if only as a symbol of the value of your work and the privacy you expect. You're going to be penning events, thoughts, suppositions, theories, relationship problems, fantasies, and other commentary that might be misunderstood by family members or friends or that might embarrass you at a time when you least need more aggravation in your life. But we've never seen locking diaries with pages big enough to be useful for journaling, so we came up with an alternative: Find a secure, personal, safe place to keep your journal away from prying eyes and hands. If you feel you need it, buy a lock box at a stationery store. You can store your book in the box, to keep private any notes you've written on its pages.

Resist the urge to use a loose-leaf binder. This journal will become a permanent reference manual, especially during the weeks when you are most intensely fighting fibromyalgia. It's better not to shuffle or remove pages. It's a form of self-censorship of "unacceptable" thoughts that perfectionists and goodists are adept at. If you leave your notes in their original order, you can review your progress and see their evolution. What's troubling you now may be an emotion much more deeply seated than what troubled you some weeks ago. You may see a change in how you feel about past anger or grief. Or you may notice that while your journal entries in Weeks One and Two concerned major problems, by Week Five you're stretching to find new troubles to write about. Some journalers find the opposite: They attack and deal with superficial things early on, and later they steel their courage and confront the really tough stuff.

Use pen, not pencil. The reason, again, is to make your journal entries both candid and permanent. Feel free to change or cross out words and even whole sentences; just don't scribble over the words so much that you can't read them, because changes themselves may be significant. Deciding, for instance, to change the word *surprised* to *horrified* shows how far you've come in acknowledging your strong emotions.

Some of us write so seldom in longhand, we've almost forgotten how. Some of us start with such pains in our hands or fingers, we can't hold a pen for very long. If you need to start your journal on a computer, be sure not to edit anything you write. A nifty way to cut down the temptation to edit, which is so easy in most software, is to stick to the bare-bones writing software that comes with Windows or Macintosh. In Windows it's called WordPad; it has no automated editing or spell-checking tools. Switch to the bound ledger book and ballpoint pen as soon as your health permits. If you're uncomfortable holding ordinary hard ballpoint pens, try a pen with a soft or cushioned barrel.

JOURNAL METHODS

Journaling is simple. In fact, the simpler you keep it, the better it'll work against fibromyalgia. You just write what's on your mind, then read what you wrote. By seeing what's on your mind, in new detail or in a new context, you can often locate festering anger, accept that it's triggering the rage that's behind your symptoms, reflect on it, and, in doing so, dump both it and the painful biochemicals it generates out of your system.

The exercises we'll assign will help you focus on all the sources of anger, grief, or shame in your life. Be careful that you don't just go through the motions. This is therapy, pure and simple, so bring to it as much enthusiasm as you can and as positive and confident an attitude as possible. Stay thoughtful, but don't get literary. We're looking for clarity, not literary merit.

Our goal in journaling is to open a mental pathway from what's at the top of your mind down toward something that's been buried in the dungeon of stuff you'd just as soon forget about. To help you do that—to keep your mind focused on areas that we've found to be maximally worthwhile for fibromyalgia sufferers—we've provided specific tasks for you in the Assignment Scheduler in Chapter 10. We'll also have you make journal entries about things you've discovered in the Relationship Planner (in Chapter 4) and My Past, Present, and Fibromyalgia-Free Future (also in Chapter 4).

Whenever you start a journaling assignment, do the following:

○ *Warm up* by reflecting, for a quiet five minutes, on what you will be writing in your journal. For some days, we have scheduled specific topics. On other days you need to pick your own topic.

○ *Realize that you can write about anything*, with this exception: Do not write about your physical fibromyalgia symptoms, or you'll be feeding your illness instead of starving it out. Writing about, even thinking about fibromyalgia symptoms helps your brain trick your body into feeling fibromyalgia. Remember, the physical symptoms are created to distract you from noticing painful emotions. Take command. Don't get distracted!

○ *Start a new page for each entry.* If you sit down to journal twice in one day, start each journaling session on a new page. That way you can easily review any attitude changes.

○ *Date the starting page* on the first line. Also enter the time.

○ *Choose a topic.* On the second line, write down in a few words what you think you'd like to write about next. It could even be something like "Why didn't I start this sooner?" or "I can't believe all I've accomplished today" or "Boy, do I have some complaints to deal with."

○ *Leave the next line blank* for now, so that you can revisit the topic later.

○ *Now write about your feelings* connected with this topic, in plenty of emotional detail. Be willing to dig deep. If the feelings associated with a recent event remind you of a past event, then write about that too. Remember, this is for you. You'll be the only one ever to read what you're writing. If you're stuck for what to say about your feelings, answer the who-what-when-where-how-why questions on page 141. This is jour-naling, not journalism, but answering those six basic questions can help prod old memories. Who besides you played a starring role, and who played a supporting role? What happened? When did it happen? Where? How did it play out, and how did it end—or hasn't it ended yet? Most important, why do you think it ended up with you angry, upset, frustrated, or sad?

○ *Contemplate.* After you've covered a topic, reflect for five minutes on what you just wrote and on the situation that prompted the journal entry. If you don't want to because it's too painful, too embarrassing, or whatever, just let yourself feel what you can about your reaction to what you wrote and use that as information for future reference. A desire to avoid even thinking about a certain topic or memory is a sure-fire clue that it is emotionally rich and may be a source of symptoms for you.

○ *Revisit the topic.* Go back to the blank right under your first topic line. Now write what the situation was really about. What you write down once your mind is freed is often quite different from what you first wrote. Notice the differences in the example on page 157.

○ *Revisit the journal entry.* If your journaling led you down a path somewhat different from the one you thought you'd follow, see if you find significance in the difference between what you chose for your initial one-line description of your topic and what you wrote later, after contemplation. Then go to the end of this journal entry, leave a line blank, and write a short explanation of what the key differences were and why you believe they occurred.

You needn't limit your journaling to the assignments or blocks of time on your schedule. If you encounter a hairy problem or go through an epiphany or have a sudden insight, by all means, grab the journal and write. But stick to the format used in assigned journal entries.

Your journal writing is not going to make *The New Yorker*. It's not supposed to interest anybody but you. You'll be wasting your time if you polish your phrases. You'll get no good marks—not here, anyway. Don't rewrite to get your facts straight; in fact, there could be meaning in getting the facts wrong. If the details come to you easily, fine. If not, write what you remember. If you hit a fuzzy patch, it's just as useful to write what might have occurred. Sometimes it's the perception of an event, not the event, that causes emotional pain.

If you suddenly get an urge to change something you wrote, that's okay. Draw a line through the old passage and write the new material just above. Remember, you should still be able to read both versions. That's why we recommended that you invest in a wide-ruled notebook or double-space what you put down. Later you'll reread your journal entries, and one task will be to make sense of these changes.

SAMPLE JOURNALING ENTRY

Topic: More humiliation in the office

Revisited topic: *I didn't swallow my anger again*

The first thing I see when I go into John's office is that humiliating pinup of Marilyn Monroe on the wall. I feel like I'm in a locker room, not an office. John barks, "What do you want?" I feel like a child. I bring him the memo to sign, but he meets me halfway and grabs my behind as usual. I wriggle away, but he thinks I'm wriggling because I love it. I hand him the memo, but now he's caressing my rear. I think what he said was, "You got it, flaunt it." I turned beet red, and I could feel the pain starting in the back of my neck. I tried to get his attention back to the memo by saying, "Mr. Johnson needs you to sign this memo after you've checked it over." But he breathes down my stiffening neck and says, "If you checked it over, I won't get in hot water, right?" That got me really angry. I finally got up the nerve to say, "I'm not getting paid to know what Mr. Johnson wants." He finally saw that I was angry, let me go, and signed it. As I was on my way out, he asked me to refill his coffee cup. I ignored him as if I hadn't heard him. But of course eventually I got him the coffee, only I put it on his desk when he was out of the office. Twice in one day was too much.

You know, this is not about my humiliation. It's about finally getting angry about the way John treats me and showing some of that anger. Next time, instead of feeling humiliated, I think I can get angry right out at John for trying to humiliate me. That's a much more appropriate response.

JOURNALING ASSIGNMENTS

In the Assignment Scheduler (Chapter 10), we'll allot time for journaling just about every day. It's important to perform all of the assigned writing—if possible, at the assigned period. However, if there's more on your mind that you want to write about in your journal at the same time, do so. You know yourself best—and will come to know yourself better and better—so if you think something is appropriate for your journal, it is.

THE FIBROMYALGIA TIME LINE

The following charts can help you find significant insights into sources of emotional events or trauma that contributed to, and still contribute to, your fibromyalgia. In the Historical Record of My Key Milestones, opposite, fill in the called-for dates. Try to get the years correct without spending a lot of research time. It's okay to approximate the months. Later on, if you find that more precise dates are important to some link you wish to explore, you may want to pick others' brains or go through family albums to refine particular dates. When finished, follow the instructions for My Fibromyalgia Time Line on page 161. Remember, reflecting on the emotional impact of each of these events is the most important aspect of this exercise, It requires as much concentration as you can muster.

HISTORICAL RECORD OF MY KEY MILESTONES

My pet name for my fibromyalgia:

Event	Approx. month	Year	Emotional impact rating on a scale of 0–10 (0 = most pain, 10 = most pleasure)
My birth			
Earliest event I can recall			
Graduation from high school			
Graduation from college			
Marriage(s)			
Birth(s)			
Separation(s)/divorce(s)			
Death of father			
Death of mother			
Death of a sibling (name)			
Death of significant person(s)			
Highly negative event in my life (not elsewhere specified on this chart)			
Highly negative event in my family (not elsewhere specified)			
Fibromyalgia probably started			
Fibromyalgia diagnosed			
Major accident(s) or trauma(s) involving me (name the event)			

(continued)

HISTORICAL RECORD OF MY KEY MILESTONES

Event	Approx. month	Year	Emotional impact rating on a scale of 0–10 (0 = most pain, 10 = most pleasure)
Major accident(s) or trauma(s) involving family members (name the event and family member)			
Major illnesses involving me (name illnesses)			
Major illness involving family members (name the illness and family member)			
Start of major job(s)			
Ending date of job(s) I quit			
Date I was fired from job(s)			
Other significant events (describe)			

Now, referring to the record above, enter significant events in My Fibromyalgia Time Line, opposite, in chronological order. Circle in red the row that contains the entry for when you probably started showing signs of fibromyalgia. Study the time line for possible relationships that you or your doctor(s) may not have recognized before. Later we will assign journaling that relies on data and correlations presented in this chart.

MY FIBROMYALGIA TIME LINE

Event	Approx. month	Year	Emotional impact rating on a scale of 0–10 (0 = most pain, 10 = most pleasure)

TALK TO YOURSELF

In addition to journaling, you can help heal fibromyalgia by talking directly to your brain as if it could hear and respond (actually, it can). You probably already do it in some form, such as, "Hey, brain, start working. I have to pick up the kids in twenty minutes!" With a little effort, we can customize this technique for your fibromyalgia-fighting arsenal. It's another way to harness your conscious mind to overpower your unconscious. It can accomplish many of the same results as meditation and journaling, but since talking can be completely internal, it's easier to do on the go.

Dr. Selfridge occasionally starts a conversation with her own mind: "I hurt. You know that I'm hurting. When I hurt, it means you've been hiding anger again. What is it now?" She has a ready list of possible aggravators to choose from, including her relationships with two daughters, one ex-husband, and a great many medical group practice administrators. While her mind skims through the list, her pain disappears on its own. She says to herself, "It's gone. Don't know which of those was the big one, but I feel better now." She says this happens every time she uses this kind of self-talk.

Cynthia learned the technique from Dr. Selfridge, and it works just as quickly for her. Whenever she feels pain, she commands her brain, "Knock it off!" If the pain persists, she figures there must be more significant anger causing it, so, as she puts it, "I go deeper." She asks her mind, "Why are you doing this to me? I have a strong body, strong mind. This should not be happening to me." Most of the time, it stops happening to her. Cynthia says she was able to turn herself around—and dump the pains of fibromyalgia—in only forty-eight hours after Dr. Selfridge introduced her to meditation, journaling, and self-talk. For her, self-talk was the most effective of the three.

Check out some of these self-talk statements and use them or make up your own.

"Hey, Brainiac, I know what you're up to. This is TMS and I'm not gonna be fooled."

"I know that this pain is emotion trying to find a way out. I know that it is temporary, benign, and reversible. I can do anything I want."

"I wonder what big, bad hairy emotion is so incredibly important right now in my subconscious mind that it requires this physical symptom as a distraction."

"Okay, my neck hurts. What is it this time? Rage, anger, fear, grief? I don't know for sure but it has to be one of those to hurt this badly. I wonder."

"WOW. I'm tired. Something emotional must be up. Wonder what it is?"

Voicing your commands out loud enhances their power and immediacy, but if you're around other people, you can say them in your head. Whatever you tell yourself, mean it. Don't make promises to yourself that you won't or can't keep. Your unrealized expectations of yourself may come back to haunt you as grief or shame.

You may be surprised that self-talk can work so well and quickly. Remember, any thought or belief that you have involves a chemical change in your brain. Change your thoughts and the beliefs behind them, and you change your brain chemistry. We already know that changing your brain chemistry changes your body response. What this means is that you can heal through words.

VISUALIZATION

Visualization is a popular tactic these days with many professional motivational gurus. They teach salespeople and football players how to visualize making that big sale or game-winning touchdown. Just as they use it to improve their performance, we can use it to improve our health. In it, you meet your emotions at the door of your unconscious by changing both your emotions and your unconscious into concrete images.

While self-talk is quite literal and left-brained, like journaling, visualization is more right-brained, or symbolic. Instead of using words to address your brain, make a realistic or symbolic picture of the pain-causing problem. If you're comfortable with realism, try to see with your mind's eye the person or situation causing the anger. If you prefer symbols, picture the emotion as a pig, a jackass, a devil, a mountain—something you can relate to and act on. Once you've pictured the cause of the problem, try to visualize a solution. Whether it's realistic or symbolic doesn't matter; what's important is to imagine yourself getting rid of it. Kick the jackass or blow up the mountain in your mind's eye. Make a movie of it. Watch it happen. Allow yourself to feel satisfaction at the ending that makes you happy.

Georgia learned visualization from a pain clinic psychologist. But it didn't entirely relieve her pain until Dr. Selfridge explained the dynamics of fibromyalgia. Once she understood what her repressed emotions were doing, she could visualize herself to health. When new pain hits—even briefly—she visualizes an ugly rock next to a calm pond. She has that image ready in her mind, so it takes only a microsecond to pop it vividly into place. Once it's there, all she does is reach out and toss the rock as far as she can into the water, and the pain is gone. She still uses symbolic visualization frequently, and figures she'll be using it to stay healthy the rest of her life.

Dr. Selfridge imagines her emotions as a naughty monster that she seeks out in the deep, dark forest of her unconscious mind. The monster insists on hide-and-seek, so she never finds it—but her symptoms go away nonetheless.

If you used symbolic visualization, what image would you choose to be your personal counterpart of Georgia's rock and Nancy's monster? How would you act on that image to get rid of your pain? Try it. Savor the way it makes you feel. You slay the dragon every time.

Experiment now with all the techniques you've learned in this chapter:

○ In your journal, write commands to yourself for trimming yesterday's biggest anger down to size.

○ Talk to yourself out loud using whatever style you normally use in your journal. See if you can self-talk about these longer and more complex problems.

○ Visualize and draw in your journal (or describe in words if you can't draw) a realistic-looking picture or series of pictures showing how a past anger-, grief-, or shame-causing event made you feel.

○ Visualize and draw (or describe in words) a symbolic picture or series of pictures showing the event just mentioned, or another strong emotion you felt recently.

While some former fibromyalgia sufferers use self-talk and visualization to great effect, we haven't scheduled them extensively, because they are sometimes slower to show results than meditation and journaling in the initial push to rid yourself of fibromyalgia. But once you feel comfortable using these other tools, we suggest that you spontaneously use one or both every time the need arises, not just during your formal recovery sessions.

TIME FOR JOURNALING, SELF-TALK, OR VISUALIZATION

There will be days when you are especially sore, tired, ornery, or out of sorts. Keep doing your journaling, meditation, and other assignments on those days. On the very days when your spirits are lowest, you may make your biggest breakthroughs. Hang in there and get well.

While we're actively working to root out your fibromyalgia, it's important to stick as closely as possible to a schedule that lets you bring your maximum energy to all the assigments. We've recommended two work sessions daily. Get used to writing in your journal during one or both sessions. There's nothing wrong with changing the schedule around a bit; just be sure you put in all the required time on each appointed day—no matter what.

REVISIT YOUR JOURNAL

At the end of each week:

○ Reread the week's journal entries

○ Make notes with red pen about your possible motives for any changes you made

○ Mark in red circles the places where you now believe you should have been angry, but didn't show it

○ Mark with red underlines any words or phrases that suggest anger, such as:

bark	clobber	flatten
bash	destroy	hit
blast	dirty	kick
blow up	disgrace	scream
bomb	dump on	sock
burst	explode	yell
bust		

Summarize these observations for each day's journal entry. What kinds of changes did you make? Is there a pattern to them? Did you make changes that sharpen your point of view? Did the changes soften your initial attitude? Were you tougher on other people the first time or the second? Are you tougher on yourself the first time or the second? Why? This is marvelous food for journaling thought.

As part of each week's wrap-up session, consider each underlined red anger indicator and note whether it's clear now why the anger went underground. In singling out and analyzing each provocative incident, did you learn anything that might be helpful in the future? Can you take away any one-word or one-line bits of wisdom to help you remember and use what you learned?

Next consider each circled portion. You've identified a situation where you ought to have been angry. In fact, you probably were angry, but only under the surface, which means you buried the anger in your subconscious, where it became more dangerous to your health. Even once you're free of fibromyalgia, you'll want to keep a sharp eye out for the kinds of situations that you circled, and make sure you defuse the anger before it triggers something in your subconscious. Make a habit of examining these circled situations whenever you experience even minor fibromyalgia symptoms.

While revisiting each week's journal entries, dwell some on your favorite warm and fuzzy recollections. Life is way too short not to take pleasure whenever the opportunity presents itself—and being happy stirs your healthful hormones. For each of these weekly journal revisitations, spend the final fifteen minutes examining and chronicling the happier memories.

REVISIONIST JOURNALING

At the end of each week, reassess your progress. If what you've been doing with your journal so far is working for you, carry on. By "working," we mean either that you have discovered strong feelings you weren't aware of before and are starting to develop tools for coping with what you're finding, or that regularly looking for those feelings has chased away some of your symptoms.

If you haven't noticed any change yet, you might want to add revisionist journaling. It could make the difference. (Even if you're feeling better, you may want to add it to your arsenal.)

Here's what to do: Choose a topic. Spend five to ten minutes skimming the week's journal entries, especially the places where you highlighted anger words with red underlines and circled spots where you could have expressed anger, and choose one of these as a topic. If you can't find big, juicy examples of anger, either expressed or suppressed, comb through everything you wrote in your journal last week and pick what still frustrates you the most.

Date the next empty left-hand page in your journal and write "Unrevised" at the top, followed by your topic. Leave the next line blank except for a number from 1 to 10, your Frustration Index for either right now or when you first jotted the entry in your journal. (Below you'll find a chart of definitions for each level of the Frustration Index.)

FRUSTRATION INDEX

1 Feeling good, really good

2 Life is going well

3 Life is going okay

4 I don't feel much anger at all

5 I'm angry enough to want to get out of the situation now

6 I'm angry enough to clench my fists and/or grit my teeth

7 I'm angry enough to hear my heart pump and feel my face get red

8 I'm frustrated to the point of not being able to think straight

9 I'm ready to punch a hole in the nearest wall

10 I'm ready to grab a brick and do damage

Now imagine you're going to shoot a short video of the event you've selected. Outline the event as it actually happened, or as it happened according to the entry you made in the journal. Include enough details so anyone can see it happen: "John's office, where a revealing pinup of Marilyn Monroe hangs cockeyed on one wall.

Jane enters. John gets up from chair, moves quickly to Jane, loudly barks, 'What do you want?' and reaches around Jane to grab her fanny."

On the opposite page, write the date, "Revision," and a new description of the topic. Make the new topic subjective, upbeat, triumphant. If you're at a loss for words, just add "I win this time" to the original topic.

Now, scene by scene or line by line, rewrite the script to give it a happy outcome. You are the writer and director. This is fiction. Make your characters behave the way you'd like them to, and alter the set to your liking. You can even turn the drama into comedy so long as in this version you win absolutely, hands down, no doubt about it. You can skunk or slaughter the bad guy. You can run a mile in three minutes. You can fly. We impose only two rules: You triumph, and you don't include your symptoms in the rewrite.

Here's how you might rewrite the above example, starting just after John shoves his paw at you. "I twist to dodge his grabby hand, and smoothly shove Mr. Johnson's memo to where he'll wrinkle it up before he connects with my skirt. He sees Johnson's name on the memo, so he stops cold. (Johnson is a real stickler for neatness, even for in-house memos.)

"I tell him, 'Mr. Johnson needs you to sign this memo after you've checked it over.'

"John says, 'Have you checked it over? If I sign it you guarantee that I'm not going to get in hot water, right?"

"I tell him, 'I checked it but I'm not privy to what Johnson wants. That's your job.'

"John protests, 'Not true. That's why we have great-looking girls—to keep us happy and out of trouble.'

"John's eyes are not on the memo, but on where his left hand is usually firmly anchored to my rear. He says, 'You got it, baby, you ought to flaunt it. Nothing to be ashamed of, is it? It's a work of art. Two works of art, really.'

"John manages to scrawl his name on the document and, as he hands it to me, he pats me a couple of times and says after me, 'Hey, and my coffee mug just ran out of java.'

"I turn around and tell him with a big grin, 'You won't be needing coffee anymore. You just OK'd Mr. Johnson's memo that fired you today without notice or severance pay. Bye, loser.' "

Quickly reassess your frustration, giving it a new number between 1 and 10. If it isn't at least two points lower, revise the script again. This time really indulge your fantasies. If you think you didn't feel any anger, grief, shame, or frustration, make up some and get it onto the page!

What's all this playacting about? It's to realize that you needn't actually fight out a troubling situation in order to confront your hidden emotions. It's a safe way to deal with anger so piercing you couldn't show it when it happened, to let off the steam that's been boiling ever since, to stop it from feeding your fibromyalgia. If this is what it takes, keep on revising. With practice, you'll imagine anger away so quickly, it can become automatic, like reaching up and pushing a strand of hair out of your eyes.

Remember, in confronting anger this way, you're not passing judgment on whether the trigger of that emotion is right or wrong, moral or immoral, ethical or unethical, or on whether you or the other guy is a good person or a louse. After all, you don't pass judgment when you grab an aspirin for a headache. Putting the feeling in its place is your goal. Reflecting on it in every way imaginable is sufficient. You are still a free person able to make moral and ethical judgments. Our methods change nothing at all about your sense of right or wrong, or about your ability to engage in debates, arguments, decision making, or anything else. All you're doing is spending time acknowledging what drives fibromyalgia into your body—and, more important, what drives fibromyalgia out of your body.

Whatever you can do, or dream you can, begin
it. Boldness has genius, power, and magic in it.
—Johann Wolfgang von Goethe

9 PUT YOUR DREAMS TO WORK

By now we hope that we've convinced you that
the end of fibromyalgia lies in your hands—as
well as in your heart, your head, and every other
part of you, internal or external, mental or physical. Although we think of our bodies, brains,
and minds as separate parts, they work as one
and meet the world as one. Small wonder, then,
that many medical scientists and physicians
advise us to pay attention to our dreams. They're
windows through which we can see what's
going on deep within our bodies.

In his many books Deepak Chopra points to
dreams as signals of overall health. Biochemist
Candace Pert includes significant data about
dreams in her book *Molecules of Emotion*.

WHERE DO DREAMS COME FROM?

Dr. Pert explains that when a person dreams, the mind and body work together like a network, "retuning itself each night for the next day."[50] She adds that during a dream, "different parts of your bodymind are exchanging information, the content of which reaches your awareness as a story, complete with plot and characters drawn in the language of your everyday consciousness."

This whole-body retuning that occurs during our dreams involves an unbelievable number of electrical and chemical processes. In one, the neuropeptides, the messenger molecules that carry information and emotions, "spill out into the system . . . and bind to receptors to cause activities necessary for homeostasis, or return to normalcy." While the body works at returning all of its sensitive circuits and chemical processes to optimal condition, "information about these readjustments enters your consciousness in the form of a dream, and since these are the biochemicals of emotion, that dream has not only content but feeling as well."

Dr. Pert explains how dreams can help us toward freedom from fibromyalgia: "Strong emotions that are not processed thoroughly are stored at the cellular level. At night, some of this stored information is released and allowed to bubble up into consciousness as a dream." Letting those emotions into our consciousness and then dispatching them, Dr. Pert says, is what helps us get well. "Capturing that dream and reexperiencing the emotions can be very healing, as you either integrate the information for growth or decide to take actions toward forgiveness and letting go."[50] Fibromyalgia sufferers' bodies feel the pain of biochemicals released by our emotions, unprocessed anger in particular, so dreams are specific opportunities to do this needed processing.

Most people dream in symbols, which are just hints about the fears and situations that provoked intense feelings. But sometimes a dream cuts right to the message. A patient in Dr. Selfridge's family practice, who normally paid little attention to her dreams, came in for a routine physical exam and asked for a blood sugar evaluation. Dr. Selfridge asked why, since the patient had no symptoms of the disease, no family history of the illness, and no risk factors for it. The patient said she'd dreamed the night before that she was diabetic. Dr. Selfridge ran the test and, sure enough, it found diabetes.

Many of Dr. Selfridge's fibromyalgia victims say at first that they don't dream. In truth, we all dream, but some of us don't consciously recall the dreams after waking up. Often it's because our dream dredges up a repressed emotion we've made ourselves forget. Some of us learned young to forget our dreams because they frightened us enormously early in life. Most of us can reacquire the knack of remembering what we've dreamed—although first you may need to convince yourself that, as an adult, you can handle what terrified you as a child.

HOW TO START HARNESSING YOUR DREAMS

A few simple techniques can help you harness your dreams to help heal fibromyalgia.

○ Decide firmly that from now on you will write down all key episodes in each night's dreams.

○ Decide that you will do this every time you wake up, whether that's in the morning or in the middle of the night.

○ Set your journal on a nightstand or chair next to your bed. (If for reasons of privacy you don't want to do this, buy another notebook just for recording your dreams.)

○ Set two pens next to the journal (one for when the first inevitably runs out of ink).

Decide, before getting into bed, that you are going to remember your dreams tonight. If necessary, use self-talk to convince yourself it can happen.

○ As you drift off to sleep, think about something pleasant that you'd like to dream about. (If you tend not to remember your dreams, make yourself visualize this dream happening.)

○ When you wake up, reach immediately for your pen and journal. Jot down whatever comes to mind, whether or not it seems like you're writing about a dream. Even if you just remember a few scenes or one emotion, immediately write what you recall. If you remember nothing, make something up—the first thing that comes to mind is probably related to what you were dreaming about.

Each day you'll find yourself getting a little better at remembering your dreams.

If you feel you need more help unlocking your dreams, read *Exploring the World of Lucid Dreaming,* by Stephen LaBerge and Howard Rheingold. It's like a cookbook, with many different recipes to start you dreaming.

WHAT TO DO WITH YOUR DREAMS

A note of caution: After you make your first move toward freedom from fibromyalgia, you may dream more vividly. At first it could seem frightening, even if you're not afraid of your dreams. At this stage of healing, you are starting to dredge up some anger, and it finds its way into your dreams. Confronting such unpleasant emotions is no fun, even in a dream.

As patients move closer to wellness, their dreams tend to become less threatening. Maybe they're more comfortable with their emotions. Maybe there are fewer threatening incidents and people left to encounter. Still, dreams are a healthier, more acceptable outlet for the subconscious than physical symptoms—so let them come!

Glenda is an example. She knows well what it's like to have scary dreams. Even after she got well, she kept having threatening dreams. But now that she's learned to expect them, she treats them as tools—similar to a physical fibro spot—to help keep her fibromyalgia-free. She advises others, "After every dream, but especially the scary ones, examine what scared you. Did an enemy pursue you? Which enemy?" Once she can put a name or a face on the enemy, Glenda finds it easy to cut the threat down to size.

For many people, writing down their dreams in detail is sufficient to dissipate the problematic emotions that drive them. Other people need to work hard to keep from censoring what they remember, especially erotic, violent, or very dramatic dreams. If you're having trouble overcoming self-censorship, keep reminding yourself that it's the dreams that are talking to you, not the other way around. Become a reporter. Write down what the dreams say, not what your inhibitions dictate.

Once you've written down what you remember in as much detail as possible, read what you wrote. Your dreams may be speaking in symbols, abstractions, or parables, so look deeply. An erotic dream may not really be about sex. An embarrassing dream may be less about an incident than an attitude. See if you can figure out what they really mean to you. If you can't, don't sweat it; just letting the matter sift through your brain is often all the attention you need to give it. We're not performing brain surgery here, just putting all the possible tools at your disposal.

Don't think that your dreams have to be dramatic or scary to be useful as tools. Sometimes the most mundane dreams can point you toward some important emotion or need. Try to get past the details to see if something with more meat on it is hiding down there. But recognize that there are also "housekeeping" dreams that mean nothing except that your body and brain are moving molecules around to get ready for their next day of work.

HOW TO SEED YOUR DREAMS

Once you get turned on to the art of watching your dreams, you can use them to help guide you back through healing. You can do that by deliberately structuring the subjects of your dreams. Glenda finds dreams so important, she considers them "messages from God sobering me up, telling me the way things are." She relies on them for major insight, and gives God a hand by preparing herself so she can dream about subjects she feels need investigation. Often she does this by rebuilding some part of her history: "What if I'd done this? What if I'd done that?" she wonders as she goes off to sleep. Rewriting incidents from her past is one way that Glenda seeds her dreams.

Dream seeding is surprisingly logical. It's done like this: As you get ready for bed, start thinking about a person, place, or incident that you'd like to dream about. As you crawl into bed, consider a couple of tangible components that might pop up in the dream. Don't try to write a script; simply visualize who or what you want to be there with you. If the location is important, visualize where the dream should be. Be sure pen and journal are within reach before you fall asleep.

Eventually you may want to seed your dream with a great many keys. But for your first dream-seeding experiences, try just two or three.

Using dreams to gain insight that might help guide you through life is probably like nothing you've ever done before. There are few rules, and no outsiders involved. Because you are taking charge of your own treatment, you don't have to put your trust in any stranger. You just have to trust yourself.

Hilda remembers that it took some time for all this to make sense. "I just thought the whole idea of emotions causing physical symptoms was kind of silly. I didn't think I was angry at anyone." But she decided to give our program for healing a try. "Then one evening after a phone call, I realized I was angry at this person I love. And that night I had another of my reoccurring nightmares—only I realized in the morning that it was centered around this very person. I suddenly became aware that whenever we talked to each other for a long while, I had this dream that night."

Shortly after, Hilda tried the technique of seeding her dreams. She thought about the bad dream before going to sleep, and changed the ending so it came out the way she wanted it to. She reports, "For the first time I was able to make the dream have a positive outcome. I woke up freed of the really icky feeling I used to have for a few days afterward. And my fibromyalgia symptoms went away."

Nancy noted that she could rely on a recurring dream of being persecuted in any number of settings when she was under pressure to perform, first when she was in school, especially around exam time. The dreams continued, though less frequently, when she transitioned into her medical practice. She decided to journal her dreams when she read that they might provide some insight into her subconscious mind. The journaling actually worked to fuel more memories of dreams. Then, if she thought about a problem before falling asleep, whether it was a relationship issue or even a diagnostic dilemma with one of her patients, and if she asked specific questions about the problem, such as "What might this illness be? What can I do to figure this out?," then frequently her dreams would contain clues, answers, or at least partial answers.

Recently, Nancy was frustrated by the fact that, in her mountain bike excursions, she just could not master the technique called "bunny hopping" to get over roots, rocks, and logs. One night, before falling asleep, she thought about the technique and wondered how her body might master it, in an attempt to seed a dream that might help her. She remembers dreaming "all night long" about hopping up and down stairs on her mountain bike, in her house, on the Spanish Steps in Rome, up the steps to the top of Water Tower Place in Chicago. The next day she just knew that she must know how to "bunny hop." She got on her bike and rode up the street, hopping on and off the curb—in perfect form.

We believe that your dream work, meditation, and journaling collaborate to thwart your fibromyalgia. They demonstrate your acceptance of the fact that your physical symptoms are being triggered by chemicals of emotion. You spend time every day thinking about these emotions in a structured, focused way, leaving little time to think about how to cope with your body's symptoms. That sends a clear message to your brain that you will no longer be distracted from emotions by your physical symptoms, and you prove it every day. Your symptoms no longer have a reason to exist, so they vanish!

THE FIVE-WEEK

PLAN TO HEAL

FIBROMYALGIA

The doctor has been taught to be interested not
in health but in disease. What the public is
taught is that health is the cure for disease.

—Ashley Montagu

WEEK ONE: PLAN TO 10 HEAL FIBROMYALGIA

We've explained what's happening in your mind-
body system to cause your suffering. We've given
you the tools and techniques to start your recovery. We've provided an overview of what you'll
cover in the treatment weeks ahead. Now we
can guide you through scheduling the specific
assignments in our program that can take you all
the way to freedom from fibromyalgia.

TIPS FOR SCHEDULING YOUR EMOTIONAL WORKOUTS

At first, plan on five weeks for your recovery
treatments. Set aside two separate hours each
day. If you work or go to school, we suggest you
schedule one session before going to work.

Many people find it's best to schedule the first workout for before you start the often-hectic routine of eating, dressing, finding things, and getting out of the house. If you stay at home, your best morning time might be shortly after the last major distraction is out of the way, such as the last child put on the bus or tucked in for a nap.

The best time for the day's second session is often the hour before your regular bedtime. Another time to consider is late in the afternoon, after work or school but before the evening meal.

Be sure your partner or any family members know that you are discussing serious business with your brain and body and they are not to disturb you for anything short of an emergency.

TIPS FOR STAYING FOCUSED DURING SESSIONS

This first week is critical to your recovery. The attitudes and intensity you apply here are likely to set the tone for your entire treatment. If you believe this is not your most important job right now—that other aspects of your life have first call on you—you'll lose your focus on getting well. We have seen several fibromyalgia sufferers who were focused on healing themselves turn their lives around in a matter of days. Those who let school, work, or relationships take first priority delayed recovery by months or more.

Don't equate focus with the number of hours you

sit meditating or writing in your journal. Some people found out that they could put in a half hour each session instead of an hour and still heal themselves in a few weeks. The trick is to approach your recovery sessions single-mindedly, putting aside every thought and concern but those directed by your assignment chart. Turn off the phone or unplug it if you need to. Turn off the cellular phone and beeper. Take off your watch and put it where you can't see it. Fill your stomach beforehand. If noises from other members of the household are likely to distract you, turn up the neutral background music. Especially during this first week, give yourself the maximum chance of achieving freedom from fibromyalgia.

Don't extend any session to more than an hour. If you want more time, add another session that day. If after two weeks of treatment you find you can't concentrate completely for sixty minutes at a time, try setting your alarm for forty-five-minute sessions. But never pare your program to less than two thirty-minute periods each day—and make the sessions this short only if you're starting to see good progress. If you decide to shorten your sessions, write the new schedule on your Assignment Scheduler (page 194). It will help keep you focused on your goal.

Use the Scheduler to plan your main activities for the five weeks. In some weeks we give more specific details based on goals we want to emphasize in that week.

WORK YOU SHOULD COVER DURING WEEK ONE

Monday A.M.: Give your fibromyalgia a name (see page 82). Also write it at the top of the Historical Record of Key Milestones, in Chapter 8, and inside the front cover of your journal.

Monday A.M. *and* P.M., *Tuesday* A.M.: Focus all of your energies on recovering from fibromyalgia. It's very important, and for some people this requires conscious, deliberate practice. If you notice your mind drifting from your assigned task, add "Focus" in front of each item preprinted on the Scheduler. During every session from now on, keep the Scheduler near at hand to remind you how vital it is to focus on this one job: recovery.

Monday P.M.: As you read this book, it's important that you jot down questions, comments, and advice for yourself as they occur to you. If you run out of room in the book's margins, continue in your journal. Be sure to date the entry and the page it refers to.

Be sure you understand everything in this book, including your margin notes. Refer to the Resources section for more information on specific topics.

Tuesday P.M.: Using a pencil, fill in the Assignment Scheduler.

Start journaling; Chapter 8 will guide you here.

Wednesday A.M., P.M.: If you haven't already filled in the Relationship Planner (page 76), My Past, Present, and Fibromyalgia-Free Future (page 91), and My

Fibromyalgia Time Line (page 161), fill them in now. If they're already filled in, review them now.

Tuesday through Friday P.M.: To launch your formal journaling, at the end of the second meditation session on each of these days spend a quiet five minutes reflecting on what it has meant to you to have undertaken this step—your doubts and concerns as well as your hopes, plans, and good feelings. Then start writing in your journal, remembering to be specific.

Thursday A.M.: Spend time understanding insights from your answers on the Relationship Planner. It is designed to focus your attention on a major source of negative emotion, particularly the anger that leads to fibromyalgia: people in your life and how you get along with them, how you see them, how you think they see you, what tensions exist between you and them, and what they do that makes you angry. There is stress in relating, even with those we love. That stress often builds to anger. How we cope with that anger can determine whether or not we get fibromyalgia. How well and how quickly those of us who come down with fibromyalgia manage to heal it often depends on how well we compensate for the stresses and aggravations of our relationships.

In the Relationship Planner, you asked yourself whether a relationship would survive your liberation from fibromyalgia. Single out any entries in the planner where you circled "maybe" in both columns 4 and 5. If there is more than one, for this session start with the one closest to the top of the chart.

Use today's journal entry to decide why you are so uncertain about this relationship. Refer to My Fibromyalgia Time Line. (If you haven't already done so, fill it in now.) Note whether the relationship started before or after your fibromyalgia. Consider the time you probably began to feel the illness' effects, not the date it was correctly diagnosed.

In this session, try to figure out whether or not the relationship will survive your recovery from fibromyalgia. As part of that analysis, carefully assess the role this person plays in generating any of the anger or other emotions that cause your fibromyalgia. This is a vital part of your recovery program, and it helps if you assess the person and the relationship with as much detachment and objectivity as possible.

Nancy recognized that a relationship with a significant other was the source of significant distress for her. As she continued to journal about this relationship, all kinds of feelings came out, but none that she could readily experience as anger. Despite this, she kept journaling for several months. Finally, she went back and read the earliest entries and had the sudden realization that her angry feelings were thinly disguised in statements about trust issues, and concern over this person's own emotional issues.

It is not inevitable that our relationships with those closest to us are factors in our fibromyalgia pain. Some people may be magnificent helpers and may help defuse or divert our harmful emotions. But often the dynamics of a relationship that starts with a pleasant tone and two people sharing equally can change subtly over time until the cumulative changes are large and dramatic. Look for this pattern in relationships you explore during this exercise, even though it may be hard to acknowledge it.

If there were an easy answer, we'd give it to you. But there is no easy answer. If you dig diligently, your journaling may help you move closer to the emotions that create your fibromyalgia.

Now, focus on starting to feel better!

FREEDOM FROM FIBROMYALGIA ASSIGNMENT SCHEDULER

PLAN TO BEAT FIBROMYALGIA

	Monday	Tuesday	Wednesday
A.M. FOR 60 MINUTES FROM _____ TO _____	Give a name to your fibromyalgia. Write it on the inside cover of your journal. Start to reread this book, making notes in it.	Finish rereading this book. Make notes in it. Make a list of other reading and reference material you need for topics you still have trouble understanding. Arrange to get the books and other help you need, if necessary.	Fill in the Relationship Planner (page 76) in pencil.
P.M. FOR 60 MINUTES FROM _____ TO _____	Continue rereading this book. Make more notes in it. If you need more space for notes, comments, questions, etc., use your journal.	Fill in the schedule in pencil. (Details are in Chapter 4.) During the last 30 minutes, write in your journal the day's most exciting event and why it's exciting. (Details are in Chapter 8.)	Fill in Part A of My Past, Present, and Fibromyalgia-Free Future (page 91) in ink, plus items you can enter in My Fibromyalgia Time Line (page 161). Details are in Chapter 4. During the last 30 minutes, write in your journal the day's most disappointing event, why it was disappointing, and any other journal entries you find important. (Details are in Chapter 8.)

Below you'll find a partially filled-in Assignment Scheduler. Complete the rest of it, noting where and when you plan to start and end each session. And don't forget to let everyone who might distract you know your schedule, reminding them that you're not to be disturbed during those times.

Thursday	Friday	Saturday/Sunday
Evaluate the Relationship Planner (page 76). Make short notes in column 6. You will need more room, so make detailed notes in your journal. Then make a detailed journal entry about what you've learned from the Relationship Planner.	Fill in Part C of My Past, Present, and Fibromyalgia-Free Future (page 91). Fill in Part D of the same form.	Spend at least 1 hour on either day writing a journal entry about what you've learned in Week One that you will use in Weeks Two through Five to reach freedom from fibromyalgia. Also revisit your journal according to guidelines in Chapter 9, and write a journal entry about that process and what you discovered.
Fill in Part B of My Past, Present, and Fibromyalgia-Free Future (page 91). Do not look at Part A's answers. Use ink. (Details are in Chapter 4.) During the last 30 minutes, write in your journal the day's most exciting event, why it's exciting, and other journal entries. (Details are in Chapter 8.)	Reconsider answers on Chapter 4 forms. Compare your book notes to your form's answers. During the last 30 minutes, write in your journal the day's most significant event, why it was significant, and other journal entries.	

FREEDOM FROM FIBROMYALGIA ASSIGNMENT SCHEDULER

SHOW YOUR BRAIN AND BODY WHO'S BOSS

	Monday	Tuesday	Wednesday
A.M. FOR 60 MINUTES FROM _____ TO _____	Reread Chapters 3, 4, and 5 for 30 minutes. Journal for 30 minutes on things in your life that need simplification, and how you plan to simplify them.	Meditate 30 minutes. (Details are in Chapter 6.) Journal for 30 minutes on this week's goals, using answers on your Fibromyalgia Facts worksheet (page 91). (Details are in Chapters 4 and 11.)	Journal 30 minutes on meditation. (Details are in Chapters 6 and 8.) Simplify something small. (Details are in Chapter 5.)
P.M. FOR 60 MINUTES FROM _____ TO _____	Meditate 30 minutes. (Details are in Chapters 6 and 11.) Simplify something small. (Details are in Chapter 5.) For 10 minutes, try to eliminate "maybe" answers in your Relationship Planner (page 76).	Journal on relationships for 30 minutes. Simplify something small. (Details are in Chapter 5.)	Meditate 30 minutes. (Details are in Chapter 6.) Do revisionist journaling. (See the end of Chapter 8.)

Thursday	Friday	Saturday/Sunday
Meditate 30 minutes. (Details are in Chapter 6.) Journal for 20–25 minutes about how this week's simplification campaign is going. Record any emotional reactions you've noticed in yourself.	Journal on relationships for 30 minutes. (Details are in Chapter 11.) Reread any chapters that you still do not significantly agree with or understand.	Spend at least 1 hour on either day writing in your journal: For 30 minutes, write about what you've learned in Week Two that takes you closer to freedom from fibromyalgia. For 30 minutes, reread last week's journal entries and write about what insights you now find in them.
Journal for 30 minutes on significant connections you see in My Fibromyalgia Time Line (page 161). Focus particularly on your emotions. Simplify something small.	Meditate 30 minutes. (Details are in Chapter 6.) Simplify something small. Assess how well this week's assignments went. Write about the five things you simplified and how they impact on your progress.	

FREEDOM FROM FIBROMYALGIA ASSIGNMENT SCHEDULER

	Monday	Tuesday	Wednesday
A.M. FOR **60 MINUTES** FROM _____ TO _____	Do anger-focused meditation for 20–25 minutes. Focus on recent anger. (Details are in Chapters 6 and 7.) Plan in your journal to choose something major to simplify. (Details are in Chapter 5.)	Do anger-focused meditation for 20–25 minutes. Focus on recent anger. (Details are in Chapters 6 and 7.) Journal for 20–25 minutes on this week's goals, using My Past, Present, and Fibromyalgia-Free Future (page 91). (Details are in Chapter 12.)	Do anger-focused meditation for 20–25 minutes. Focus on older anger. (Details are in Chapters 6 and 7.) Journal on anger or dreams, 20–25 minutes.
P.M. FOR **60 MINUTES** FROM _____ TO _____	Reread Chapters 3, 6, and 7. For 10 minutes, try to eliminate "maybe" answers in your Relationship Planner (page 76).	Journal on anger or dreams for 20–25 minutes. (Details are in Chapters 7 and 12.) Work in your journal on simplifying something major this week.	Journal on relationships for 20–25 minutes. (See Chapters 9 and 12.) Simplify something today.

Choose A.M. or P.M. for your meditation all week.

Thursday	Friday	Saturday/Sunday
Do anger-focused meditation for 20–25 minutes. Focus on older anger. (Details are in Chapters 6 and 7.) Journal for 20–25 minutes on how you simplified your life this week.	Do anger-focused meditation for 20–25 minutes. Focus on older or newer anger. (Details are in Chapter 7.) Journal on relationships for 20–25 minutes.	Spend at least 1 hour on either day writing in your journal. (Details are in Chapter 8.) For 20–25 minutes, write about what you've learned in Week Three that takes you closer to freedom from fibromyalgia. For 20–25 minutes, reread the week's journal entries and write about what insights you now find in them.
Journal on anger or dreams for 20–25 minutes. Refine the simplification of your life that you started this week. (Details are in Chapter 5.)	Journal on anger or dreams for 20–25 minutes. Finish simplifying this week's goal. (Details are in Chapter 5.) Make a journal entry about the simplification.	

FREEDOM FROM FIBROMYALGIA ASSIGNMENT SCHEDULER

FIBROMYALGIA FREEDOM: TIME TO FEEL REALLY WELL AGAIN

	Monday	Tuesday	Wednesday
A.M. FOR 60 MINUTES FROM _____ TO _____	Meditate for 20–25 minutes. (Details are in Chapter 6.) Simplify something modest in your life. (Details are in Chapter 5.)	Remember all this week to act again as though you are feeling well. Meditate for 20–25 minutes on feeling well again or on anger. (Details are in Chapters 6 and 7.) Simplify something modest in your life.	Meditate for 20–25 minutes on feeling well again or on anger. Journal for 20–25 minutes on "emotional housecleaning." (Details are in Chapter 13.)
P.M. FOR 60 MINUTES FROM _____ TO _____	Reread at least Chapter 10 plus as much of Chapters 3, 6, and 7 as you can. Study Parts C and D of My Past, Present, and Fibromyalgia-Free Future (page 91) for new insights into what life will be like without fibromyalgia. For 10 minutes, try to eliminate "maybe" answers in your Relationship Planner (page 76).	Journal for 20–25 minutes on dreams, anger, and feeling well again. (Details are in Chapters 7, 9, and 13.) Practice your use of self-talk and visualization. This time, focus them on feeling well. (Details are in Chapters 8 and 13.)	Journal for 20–25 minutes on dreams, simplifying things in your life, or feeling well again. (Details are in Chapters 5, 9, and 13.) Simplify something modest in your life.

Schedule meditation sessions consistently for A.M. or P.M.
All this week, remember what it felt like to feel well.

Thursday	Friday	Saturday/Sunday
Meditate for 20–25 minutes on feeling well again, relationships that aren't working, or anger. Journal for 20–25 minutes on feeling well and finding regular exercise time and activities.	Meditate for 20–25 minutes on feeling well again. Journal for 20–25 minutes on dreams and relationships. Start exercising. (Details are in Chapter 13.)	Spend at least 1 hour on either day writing in your journal. (Details are in Chapter 9.) Write about what you've learned in Week Four that takes you closer to freedom from fibromyalgia. In particular, focus on feeling well again. (Details are in Chapter 10.) Reread the week's journal entries and write about what insights you now find in them. Exercise. (Details are in Chapter 13.)
Journal for 20–25 minutes on dreams, relationships, or feeling well again. Simplify something modest in your life.	Journal for 20–25 minutes on dreams, simplifying things in your life, or feeling well again. (Details are in Chapters 9 and 11.) Simplify something modest in your life.	

FREEDOM FROM FIBROMYALGIA ASSIGNMENT SCHEDULER

	Monday	Tuesday	Wednesday
A.M. FOR 30 MINUTES FROM _____ TO _____	Journal for 20 minutes on the major benefits you have gained so far in this program and what you think you still need to work on. (Details are in Chapter 14.) Focus for 10 minutes on a major part of your life to simplify this week.	For 20 minutes, plan specific methods to simplify the chosen part of your life this week. Journal for 20 minutes on how you now feel overall. (Details are in Chapter 14.)	Work on this week's life simplification project for 10 minutes. Journal for 20 minutes on anger that's still bothering you.
P.M. FOR 30 MINUTES FROM _____ TO _____	Meditate for 30 minutes. For 10 minutes, try to eliminate "maybe" answers in your Relationship Planner (page 76). Exercise. (Details are in Chapter 13.)	Meditate for 30 minutes.	Meditate for 30 minutes. Exercise. (Details are in Chapter 13.)

Thursday	Friday	Saturday/Sunday
Work on this week's life simplification project for 10 minutes. Journal for 20 minutes on pain and anger that may still be bothering you. (Details are in Chapter 14.)	Work on this week's life simplification project for 10 minutes. Journal for 20 minutes on relationships that may still bother you. (Details are in Chapter 14.)	Spend at least 1 hour on either day writing in your journal. (Details are in Chapter 9.) Write what you've learned in Week Five that takes you closer to freedom from fibromyalgia. Reread last week's journal entries and write about what insights you now find in them.
Meditate for 30 minutes.	Meditate for 30 minutes. Exercise. (Details are in Chapter 13.)	

Always do one thing less than you think you can do.

—Bernard Baruch

11

WEEK TWO: SHOW YOUR BRAIN AND BODY WHO'S BOSS

During Week Two we expect you to make one not-so-earth-shaking simplification in your life each day. That means you have to think up something to simplify, something that you don't need, don't want, and can live more at ease without. It could be as simple as getting the kids to take out the garbage when they're supposed to or finding an alternative to driving across town to buy groceries.

But you have to do more than just figure out random solutions to small hurdles. If our program is to work for you, you have to come at the assignments here as prescribed treatments. In other words, you also have to put each of the simplifications into practice. Make them work. We've made it your goal to simplify five aspects of your life this week. You can thank us later!

DETAILS ABOUT ASSIGNMENTS FOR WEEK TWO

Monday A.M.: Sit with your journal open. Isolate some parts of your life that are good candidates for simplification. Write them down in a list. Start on an empty left-hand page so you can fill two pages with ideas for simplifying your life and see them all at once.

Jot them down as they come to you. If you run out of ideas, mentally walk yourself through a typical week, day by day, hour by hour, and, if necessary, minute by minute. We hope you come up with a list that will fill at least one page in your journal.

Next, review your list. Estimate how easy each of the ideas is to implement. In front of each idea, rate it with a number from 1 to 10, 10 being tough, 1 being a no-brainer that hardly anybody would notice.

Reread your numbered list to see if you still agree with the levels of difficulty you've assigned. Make changes wherever needed.

Monday P.M.: Choose an idea from your morning's list that's a 1 in difficulty. Your meditation assignment for this afternoon is to implement this idea. Decide what you have to do and what you must ask others to do in order to jettison this complication from your life. When you've finished your meditation session, immediately start doing whatever it takes to make it happen by the end of the day.

Tuesday P.M.: Choose an idea that's a 2 in difficulty. Decide what you have to do and what others have to do in order to jettison this complication from your life. Now make it happen.

Wednesday P.M.: Continue simplifying. Tackle an idea that's a 3 in difficulty. Draw up a battle plan, and win the battle before bedtime.

Thursday A.M.: For twenty to twenty-five minutes, evaluate in your journal how well your simplification assignment has gone so far. Identify and write down who and what specifically helped or hindered getting the assignments done. Go over your initial list of things to simplify. In light of your three days of experience with this assignment, decide if the items at levels of difficulty that are 4 and 5 should realistically be considered minor. If so, pick a 4 for this afternoon. If not, pick a 2.

Thursday P.M.: Continue simplifying. Tackle this morning's choice. Draw up a battle plan, and win the battle before bedtime.

Friday P.M.: Implement another minor simplification before bedtime. Also, assess in your journal how well you did on this week's assignments. Focus on the exercises' overall emotional impact. Summarize in writing what you expected to feel from the five things in your life that you should have simplified this week—and what you actually feel about them. Evaluate your reactions. Did they surprise you? Are you pleased, or do you feel guilty? Are you feeling less pressured than a week ago, or more? If the latter, do you know what's actually driving that sense of pressure, or is it hidden in your unconscious? If it's hidden, it needs to be confronted using meditation, journaling, self-talk, or visualization.

Through each of the coming weeks, we'll continue this simplification process. Hang in there. Try to avoid the tendency to make these sessions harder than they should be. Go with your first impressions and always be sensitive, even in the process of simplification, to any negative emotions that surface. In all our exercises, what's of paramount importance is creating the opportunity to search for these feelings.

Most of the world's work is done by people who
don't feel well.

—Sir Winston Churchill

12 **WEEK THREE: TEACH YOUR BRAIN
AND BODY TO LIVE WITH RAGE**

During the course of their treatment for fibromyalgia, some people start creating mental
walls. It's almost as if the mind is throwing up
roadblocks to healing. Dr. Selfridge's patients
have expressed these concerns:

o "If I follow your guidelines, I'll turn into a
terribly selfish and angry person, won't I?"

o "If the cure is that simple, how come I got
fibromyalgia in the first place?"

o "I didn't have any anger until you started
treating me. How come?"

o "You think this is all in my head? I've heard
that before and I didn't like it then either!"

No, healing your fibromyalgia won't make
you selfish or angry—but sensitive folks like us

need to know why. If you still have doubts that you have unconscious emotions like anger, go back and reread Chapter 7. Here's more ammunition for jumping past your own mental roadblock.

There was a time when adult-onset diseases of all sorts were probably a rarity, since our earliest ancestors died early—eaten by predators or smashed in a fall off a cliff while trying to kill the night's dinner. Cave paintings don't show any illnesses, and archaeologists haven't found signs of fibromyalgia in skeletons or in artifacts buried with them. During Old Testament times, if you didn't die due to crop failure, the wrath of God, Saul's soldiers, or leprosy, you may have lived disease-free—if we're to judge from what the Bible *doesn't* report. But over in ancient Greece, doctors were combating plague and other bacterial infections, and learning to fix broken bones and overextended muscles.

Our bodies and brains haven't kept up with the change from life thousands of years ago to largely indoor, mentally stressful modern life. Nowadays, as Dr. Stanley J. Sarnoff, physiologist at the National Institutes of Health, says, "The process of living is the process of reacting to stress." Now there's a new kind of illness to treat, caused or exacerbated by our modern lifestyle. Fibromyalgia is just one of the hundreds of ailments in this category, only some of which have been cataloged.

The medical community keeps looking for a cause—a bacterium or virus, a misplaced gene or two, anything tangible—to explain how fibromyalgia starts, so they can develop a cure. All they've done so far is to lengthen the list of symptoms, which they know are real because they've been able to assess patients' pain, document their sleep disturbances, and measure their levels of substance P (the neuropeptide that seems to pass the sensation of pain throughout our bodies). And, not finding a cause, some resort to saying, "It must be all in your head."

Dr. Nortin M. Hadler noted in *Spine*, a major pain journal, that whenever a new indicator is added to fibromyalgia's symptoms, doctors find more people with that indicator. He doubts we'll ever find a physical cause or causes—yet, he says, "advocates are undaunted, trying to ferret out an answer from the muscle or endocrine or nervous systems of the sufferers. The sufferers are paying a substantial price for the scientific method."

Whatever fibromyalgia's cause, doctors long tried to cure it with the same techniques that repair blood, bones, and muscle. They attacked symptoms with specific antidotes, prescribing pills for migraine headache and high blood pressure. When they found spinal abnormalities, using hypersensitive X-ray and scanner equipment, they cut and repositioned what didn't conform to "average." They prescribed narcotics for pain, antidepressants for feelings of futility, and physical therapy for constricted joints. Many doctors are still trying these old treatments for the new ailments. If you've had fibromyalgia for long, chances are you were put through some of these "cures" and symptom relievers.

But some members of the medical community are learning what chiropractors, faith healers, and acupuncturists know about pain: that it's a mind-body phenomenon, not reducible to one or the other. Hospitals are opening departments of complementary medicine that take a mind-body approach to healing and employ massage therapists, herbalists, and acupuncturists along with conventionally trained physicians. This is good news for us. It means that soon there may be doctors in all of our communities who understand mind-body medicine. Soon, we hope, anyone who hit a wall of doubt during this treatment program will be able to speak their doubt to an expert face-to-face.

DETAILS ON ASSIGNMENTS FOR WEEK THREE: ANGER-FOCUSED MEDITATION AND MAJOR SIMPLIFICATION

Monday A.M.: Start by reviewing your written schedule and modify it to accommodate whether you prefer meditating in the morning or later in the day. It's possible to meditate both times, but probably not necessary if your meditation is for the purpose of healing fibromyalgia. If you believe you need more meditating, it's better to do one longer, more intense session than two shorter, less intense ones—but don't meditate for more than an hour at a stretch. We covered details of anger-focused meditation in Chapter 7. Read it again if you'd like a review of the methods and goals.

Take out your current Anger List (page 136) and read through the entries to familiarize yourself with details of the episodes you jotted down. Be especially alert for episodes that you did not immediately recognize as anger but that the Anger Cop in you analyzed and decided to call anger. Mark these episodes in red before you begin to meditate. Keep the list close at hand.

Get yourself into your basic meditative state using the techniques from Chapter 6. To refresh your memory, turn to the summary of steps at the end of Chapter 7 or keep the book open to this page while you're working on the following assignment.

Once you're comfortably meditating, take hold, with your mind, of the first anger marked in red on your list. Remember all the details of how it happened. Visualize it happening all over again. Paint it into your mind's eye with the boldest, brightest strokes possible. Don't let guilt or considerations of fair play get in the way. This is your world. You suffered from the anger. You can paint it any way you like. You are the only person capable of curing yourself of fibromyalgia.

In as much detail as possible, re-create what you saw, heard, and felt during the anger. Feel it. Feel it again. Feel it in your gut, in your throat, in your head, hands, and heart. Don't let go of it. This time, don't let it escape your full attention while it lives.

If this piece of anger has become a part of your memory—and it has, since you jotted it onto your Anger List—you probably feel like you lost the battle, and that made you angrier. By now you may feel like you surrendered to the enemy. We're here to tell you that you can win. You can squabble, negotiate, and argue compellingly.

You can yell, hit, kick, and scratch. Do it! Don't fight fair. Don't hold back. Corner the anger. Make it give up. Make the people on the other side of this anger episode lose the argument. Humiliate them. Humble them. Bring them to their knees, literally, if that gives you satisfaction. Do whatever it takes for you to feel that this time you've won the battle that led to your anger. It doesn't matter how long ago or how recent it was, how close or how distant the other star players in this scene may be now. It doesn't even matter if the anger-dredging culprit is alive or not, sick or well, happy or crushed. This is your world. This is your anger. This is how you can learn to face up to anger and kick out of your life its fibromyalgia-causing effects.

Let's look at an example. Imagine that at work, someone quits and the work that they did is "temporarily redistributed" to you and another co-worker, while "they" are looking for someone to fill the position. You are a good worker, even on your worst days, so you do the work without complaining, but after five months have passed and there are no prospects for the position and you haven't even heard that anyone has been interviewed, you begin to get suspicious. You bring this up to your manager, checking to see what is going on, and hear that because you are doing such a great job with the extra work and not even having to work overtime to get it all done (never mind that you collapse when you get home and your muscles are screaming all of the time and you have no life outside work and you are starting to get really, truly clinically depressed), your boss might not be hiring at all for that position. Nearly in tears, you run and hide in your office until you can compose yourself. This incident comes up in your meditation. You allow yourself to express, in words, your resentment and rage for being taken advantage of in this way. How dare they treat you this way after all you have done for them? Some pay-off for being loyal! You'd like to march into your boss's office, give your notice, turn around and have him check out the mistletoe you have pinned to the waistband of your slacks! You'd like to organize an uprising of the oppressed in your workplace and, like Norma Rae, stop this insanity!

Keep at it until you feel confident that you've won this time. When you're really sure that you can put that battle behind you, put a big check mark alongside that entry in your Anger List. Remarkably, you may notice that concentrating intensely on this anger and the circumstances surrounding it has released some of your pain.

Take a few minutes to return to a relaxed, focused meditative state. Gather your energy to take on the next red item on your list. Attack it as aggressively as you did the first one. It should be a little easier this time, with less guilt and fewer hesitations. Win the argument. Slough off the insult. Return the put-down with a brilliant retort. Maneuver and manipulate and scheme and jockey the image until you win. Then put it away. Add another big check mark to your Anger List, and relax.

If you feel that you're working very hard at this process, you should probably not take on more than three or four specific anger triggers at a sitting. You can handle more when you begin to feel more resilient. At any rate, stop after working at it for half an hour. Eventually this process will become automatic and carry over to your non-meditative life. You will be able to identify and focus on your anger whenever bothersome symptoms get your attention.

Use the rest of your morning session, or part of the afternoon session, to choose something major in your life that you will simplify next. Last week (and again next week) we assigned you to simplify something not too earth-shaking each day of that week. This week we want you to focus on just one big complication in your life that, when it's gone, will have brought you a giant step toward a more serene, less frazzled existence. In other words, it'll help you to get a life, and that will help you to end fibromyalgia.

Because this step should make such a significant change in your life, we want you to use this assignment time planning it carefully. Take out your journal and use about half the time listing possible aspects of your life that could stand simplification.

You may want to simplify a relationship. This could involve family, friends, work, church, whatever. Choose this kind of simplification if in the worksheet My Past, Present, and Fibromyalgia-Free Future (page 91) you gave a family or job relationship a dismal rating. Also, refer back to the Relationship Planner (page 76) to get a more objective look at how you rated the impact various people have on your life. You may have to tell a longtime friend that her whining has got to stop, or a colleague you've worked with for years that you won't cover for him any longer when he screws up. These life adjustments qualify as major simplifications.

It's likely you'll want to explore simplifying the way at least one thing you're responsible for happens around your home. Quit being the official taxi for lessons and practices, quit acting as zookeeper for the pets, quit getting up early enough to play chef at breakfast for the whole tribe. These qualify as major simplifications.

You may want to add a big dose of fun to your life. Take out the worksheet My Past, Present, and Fibromyalgia-Free Future (page 91) and see what you jotted there early in these treatment sessions. See if something that really turns you on also qualifies as a major simplification. For instance, how about insisting on planning the next vacation to give top priority to your needs, your likes, your dislikes? We think that's major enough to qualify for this assignment.

Make at least five journal entries for possible parts of your life that you'd like to simplify in a major way. Ten would not be too many. After you've compiled the list in your journal, reread each entry. Rank them from 1 to 5 (or however many you have), but don't base the ranking on how easily the simplification could be accomplished.

Rank as number 1, the change that will have the biggest impact on your life, and so on down the line.

Next, select one simplification with a ranking in the top half of your list. Consider that choice for a few minutes. Is it likely you can begin to put it into effect within the next several days? Once implemented, is it likely to simplify a significant aspect of your life? If you have second thoughts about its significance or your ability to make the change, select another item and go through the same analysis.

If you end up rejecting all of the top candidates on your simplification list as being either too insignificant or too hard to implement, here's a very important assignment to schedule for your next journaling time, no matter what that topic was originally: Spend the entire session (and the next, if that's required) answering these four questions in writing.

o Are my expectations of life too unrealistically grand, or am I unrealistically afraid of asserting my right to having a good life?

o Who is it that determines whether or not I enjoy life?

o Who should determine whether or not I enjoy life?

o For each answer above, can I find any emotions that tip me off to what may be fueling my symptoms?

Tuesday A.M.: Unless you already assigned yourself an alternative topic after Monday's simplification asssignment, take out your journal and your filled-in My Past, Present, and Fibromyalgia-Free Future worksheet (page 91). Spend the allotted time in one of these ways:

○ Reminiscing in writing about the single most-missed pleasure that fibromyalgia has robbed from your life, and the emotions associated with it

○ Writing down your plan for recovering that specific pleasure

○ Planning to recover that pleasure starting this week

Tuesday P.M., *first part:* Review your Anger List (page 136). Then move through all the steps you still find helpful in reaching a fully meditative state—relaxing, deliberate breathing, focusing on the job at hand. Now that job is to spend another rewarding session in confronting your anger.

Write in your journal about your anger or about your dreams. Remember that as you start defeating fibromyalgia's grip on you, you might start dreaming more vividly, perhaps even dreams with some scary scenes in them. Your dreams are a safe, healthy outlet for undesirable unconscious emotions. So if you've been dreaming, write down the details and then try to figure out whether and how the dreams point toward the direction your life was taking, is taking, or ought to take. Write down, in detail, these speculations and conclusions.

If you think it's more appropriate for you to focus

on anger instead of dreams, take out yesterday's and today's Anger Lists. Mark in red the three episodes in which you were most angry. Write in your journal the details of all three incidents so that you don't forget them. Evaluate how you reacted to the anger each of the three times. Evaluate how you felt and how your fibromyalgia felt after each episode. Try to be brutally honest. Suggest how you might have handled each episode differently. Always focus your writing on the goal we've set for you: to deal with anger as it happens and to reflect on anger routinely when you notice your symptoms, so that rage cannot kick up the biochemicals that fuel your illness.

Tuesday P.M., second part: Turn your journal to yesterday's planning of the major part of your life that you will simplify this week. Look at your notes about the specific aspect of life that you chose to simplify. Now turn to a clean page and fill in the date and topic; leave the revisited topic line blank.

List the steps you have to take to make your chosen simplification happen. Whom do you have to talk to about it? Who, if anybody, will have to take on new tasks as a result of your simplification? If you stop performing a task, will that have an impact on anybody else? How does all of this make you feel?

Remember how Nancy got her kids to help meal plan, cook, and grocery shop to help buy her some more time to get well? Another aspect of this simplification was to allow them to have messy rooms and to not let it bother her. They were, after all, helping her out in a way that had much more impact on her life than their clean bedrooms would.

Now, in writing, schedule each of the steps above for a specific day, time, and place. If you're on a weekly schedule with us, today should be Tuesday. Plan to perform all of these required items by Thursday evening at the very latest. We want you to be able to know on Friday that life is simpler—but if it is absolutely necessary, use Friday to clean up the final work on that goal.

Wednesday P.M., *first part:* Journal about your relationships. Take out your Relationship Planner (page 76). For the first five minutes, reread your earlier journal entries (Week Two, Tuesday P.M. and Friday A.M.). Using a red pen, put a big R in the margin and underline key words for anything that now in any way dissatisfies you. It doesn't matter whether the dissatisfaction is from disappointment, insult, stupidity, or whatever else doesn't fit your expectations for yourself. Now, spend about ten minutes using revisionist journaling (Chapters 8 and 11) to find solutions for all the problems, complaints, and unsatisfying conclusions you just marked in red. In the remaining time, write a journal entry telling, if you can, how your most recent revisionist journal entry differs in result from the two earlier entries you studied in this assignment.

Most important: Whenever you write about yourself in the journal, focus on and write about new emotions that come up, but ignore any physical symptoms or other experiences you may be having. This is the absolute key in making these sessions help you toward health.

Other work for Wednesday and Thursday: Prepare for these sessions by carrying your Anger List with you wherever you go, to dredge up older incidents. As your mind drifts or your attention catches on something that triggers memories of times long gone, be attentive for the telltale signs of anger. Jot them down on your Anger List. Get ready to deal with them. During your meditation sessions, concentrate on remembering and banishing older angers, even as far back as early childhood. After a while you ought to find two things happening: You'll resolve each item more quickly, and you won't need to involve yourself in each scenario in as much detail.

If you're not getting the hang of this method, try revisionist journaling (see Chapter 8 and especially Chapter 11). It's a more literal, left-brained way to achieve the same effect. Our goal in these sessions is not to reconstruct anger-provoking incidents in minute detail or to magnify them. Instead, it's to help you prove two things to yourself: that you are confident that the biochemicals of emotion have been causing your symptoms, and that you are insistently restricting your thinking to the emotions themselves instead of their physical effect on your body. You are creating and honing a new habit, a new way of relating to your symptoms. You are changing your brain chemistry to get better.

Friday A.M. or P.M.: Work on new or old anger, or a

combination of both. Be sure that you resolve each anger-provoking incident, but try for speed, using as little time and energy as possible. After all, you don't want to spend an hour a day for the rest of your life slogging through anger. If you've stuck with us this far, you've got a great shot at going all the way to freedom from fibromyalgia. Good job!

CHAPTER 13

The events in our lives happen in a sequence in time, but in their significance to ourselves they find their own order . . . the continuous thread of revelation.

—Eudora Welty

WEEK FOUR: TIME TO START FEELING REALLY GOOD AGAIN

WORK YOU SHOULD COVER DURING THIS TREATMENT WEEK

○ Review this book up to this point, especially Chapters 3, 5, 8, and 9.

○ Every day this week, practice anti-anger meditation (Chapter 7) and meditation on feeling well (Chapter 6).

○ Each day this week, simplify one relatively small part of your life (covered in Chapter 5). Report on this in your journal.

○ In your journal, keep tabs on your dreams. Expect that some will be unusually vivid and perhaps even frightening. (Dreams are covered in Chapter 9, journaling in Chapter 8.)

○ Keep using your journal (described in Chapter 8) to help you analyze new emotional situations, especially those provoked by old anger.

THE MOMENT OF EPIPHANY

It's now time to focus less on ridding your life of the negative and more on getting the positive juices flowing again. You'll never be able to avoid all of life's bumps and sharp turns, but you should start building and savoring happy times. Remember life without fibromyalgia? We invite you to step off the curb and sample it again.

Some people, as they recover from fibromyalgia, experience one dramatic event that signals beyond a doubt that their life has just made a major about-face. This is their moment of epiphany. It takes many forms but, without exception, it is a very emotional moment.

As Dr. Selfridge approached freedom from fibromyalgia, her mood soared higher each new pain-free day. She bounced as she strode up and down the office corridors, exhilarated at feeling well again after twenty years. Each morning was a celebration that she awoke with no pain, each evening a celebration of another pain-free day. Convinced her wellness was going to last, she wanted to share her joy with colleagues and patients.

While Franklynn worked his way to being well, he continued his job as editor of a monthly newsletter. He was working harder than ever toward a week's vacation with his companion, Judi, in the Alps. While he sensed that the treatment was working, he didn't stop to acknowledge he was feeling better until the job's pressures were behind him. When he got to the mountains, something popped. On the first day, making an easy climb to some low-altitude scenic spots, Franklynn started to say something and suddenly found himself crying. He could scarcely talk the rest of the day without crying, elated that for the first time in over a decade, he was himself again, free of fibromyalgia.

Tears kept coming easily the whole trip, as he kept feeling the stark demarcation between the old suffocating darkness of full-body pain and the pain-free pleasure he could feel looking at the splendor of the Alpine scenery. Snowy peaks, craggy glaciers, flower-lined hiking trails, the intense blue sky—he was able to enjoy it all again with every sense, holding nothing back and fearing no awful sudden let-downs. He counts it among the most intense joys he's ever experienced.

Anna and Betsy had their epiphany together. Both patients of Dr. Selfridge, they used to meet almost weekly for support. This particular week, they met at a restaurant and had been swapping news from the "fibro front." When they realized that they had finally arrived at the wellness they'd pursued, they giggled like schoolgirls. Anna laughed so hard she bumped her water glass, some of it spilling on Betsy, but neither of them cared. They were already planning excitedly for their fibromyalgia-free lives.

The following information explains details in addition to the assignments listed in the Scheduler (page 194). Their general advice should be kept in mind the entire week as we help change your attitude from feeling ill to feeling well again.

MONDAY: REMEMBER WHAT FEELING GOOD FELT LIKE

Dr. Selfridge's patients turn from as sick as can be to as good as they ever were at an unpredictable pace. Some, like Cynthia, recover in a matter of days. Cynthia works in an art gallery and is an artist herself, so she's been aware of her very sensitive nature for a long time. Intuitively she structured her lifestyle to limit stimulation, to focus inward, and to cultivate her own creativity. Her husband, also a sensitive sort, accepts her choices and is very supportive. Perhaps these factors influenced her rapid recovery.

Dr. Selfridge took a much longer time to feel completely well—she needed months to conquer all her symptoms. Not only was her brain set up by years of medical training to ignore mind-body explanations for disease, but she'd reinforced these incorrect explanations for years in her treatment of patients. In addition, her lifestyle was exactly the opposite of Cynthia's—demanding, overstimulating, frustrating, and overwhelming all of the time. Perhaps these factors slowed her recovery.

Ultimately, it isn't important how fast or how slowly you progress. Go at your own pace, and don't feel guilty. Most of us make so many adjustments in our life to accommodate our symptoms, we may even overlook the moment we start to feel better.

From now on, as you work through the assignments in this book, start looking for clues that you're losing some of your pain. Make sure that you're not continuing the accommodations you made in the past for your fibromyalgia just out of habit. Periodically try activities you abandoned—but be absolutely sure you're resuming them out of pleasure, not need. Approach these new "old" activities with care. If they involved physical endurance, accept that you may be significantly out of condition and need to start again slowly. Accept with grace a lower level of performance or a tendency to tire more easily. Work up to your previous performance level when you're confident that you're not hurting yourself.

Begin to embrace your sensitive nature and observe how it works in your favor. Rejoice that although this nervous system of yours may have contributed to your past suffering, it also provides you with gifts of insight, compassion, responsiveness, spirituality, and creativity. Focus on your buried negative emotions, to be sure, but don't fail to celebrate all the wonderful attributes that distinguish your nature, the rich emotional meaning you derive from life, and the benefits these add to your newfound health.

To make sure you're not missing any good feelings, work today with My Past, Present, and Fibromyalgia-Free Future chart (page 91). Turn to Parts C and D, the summary and comparison that point you toward your fibromyalgia-free future.

With your red pen, note today's date alongside some passage that might be evidence of your getting better, whether you're aware of it or not. For now, bypass entries where your scoring showed the largest contrast between your pre- and post-fibromyalgia experience. Typically, when so much is at stake, the strongest emotions and the biggest conflicts are the last to release their physical grip. So first single out entries where the discrepancies are not so formidable.

If your pre-fibromyalgia memories, physical and emotional, don't immediately jump to life again, don't despair. Possibly even before you noticed your symptoms, you were chided for being too sensitive and making things hard for yourself. Almost instinctively you developed strategies to live in an insensitive world, keeping your sensitivity in check. Think of how long you were reining in your emotions—and how long you had your fibromyalgia symptoms. Now consider how long it takes to rebuild a muscle that's been six months in a plaster cast. So if there's a lag in reusing your body and emotions, don't let it become frustrating. With confidence and practice, the knack will come back. You'll soon enjoy your long-lost sense of touch and smell; you'll soon appreciate the sensitivity you tried to bury long ago. If you're one of the small minority of fibromyalgia sufferers who can't reach the feelings you shut down, psychotherapy may be useful. Don't let any thoughts of failure stop you from reaching out for additional help. You deserve it.

One way to help turn on the emotions you may have flicked off to the point where they're strange to you is to reread a diary or journal that you kept before fibromyalgia got a grip on you. In going over what you wrote back then, look for signs of what you felt like before fibromyalgia. If you don't have old writings, make a list now of a dozen good times you've enjoyed—anything from bowling to big family events to the opera. Whatever you count as fun belongs on the list. Next, identify the one or two episodes that left you with the happiest emotions. During the rest of your treatment, whenever you're feeling low or frustrated, stop and try to recapture these emotions again.

It may seem arbitrary at first, but practice feeling. Touch things with interesting textures: a shiny hood ornament, a glass bubble, heavily textured drapes. Stop and smell the flowers, the new-mown grass, the tickly mist from a fountain, waffles baking, coffee perking. Look at the buildings, people, art, and whatever else used to move you, and reach for the good feeling you used to have. Anna tells about the good feeling that swept through her when she first sat through a whole movie again without having to stand up to shake out her complaining legs.

TUESDAY: START ACTING WELL

Frequent use of self-talk and visualization can encourage healthy behavior and revive good feelings. So start acting well. Act, as in a play. Assume the pleasures of good health. Smile, to remember what it feels like to smile and to remember why we smile. Make your voice sound like a healthy person's voice.

It's totally natural for those of us saddled with fibromyalgia to develop behavior patterns that mask the pain, the embarrassment, the despair. We don't clap, even when a performer puts on a once-in-a-lifetime show, because clapping hurts the palms of our hands. We don't bend to pick up loose change we've dropped or tie shoelaces that undid themselves, because bending hurts the back and hips. We look for wheeled shopping carts with plastic-padded handles because it hurts too much to carry a few items in a basket or to grasp bare metal handles.

Franklynn remembers getting fed up with people asking him "What's the matter?" when they saw him shuffling along all bent over. One night, watching TV, he saw Paul Newman, Dustin Hoffman, and others demonstrate method acting. It gave him the idea to study how normal people walked. Then he method-acted a normal walk.

Don't confuse this kind of acting with acting stoic. If you act as though you're feeling well and happy, soon you'll feel this way for real. This is how Franklynn quickly taught himself how to walk straight again.

If you can't remember what it felt like to walk when feeling well, to climb stairs when feeling well, to hold a fork when feeling well, start acting it today. Watch somebody walk who you think feels well and then walk the same way. Walk well again. Eat well again. Climb stairs well again. Work well again. Feel the joy of being well again.

WEDNESDAY: CLEAN HOUSE EMOTIONALLY

Among the toughest feelings for people recovering from fibromyalgia to deal with are those involving their closest relationships, including parents, children, spouses, co-workers, bosses, friends, and neighbors. In a way, maintaining and repairing relationships with people close to you is much like relearning to use your feelings. But it may take more work, because feelings rely only on you, while relationships involve the needs of at least two people. During your bout with fibromyalgia, your friends and family weren't static. They grew, they changed, they got promoted or found different jobs, they learned to look at you as a person in need. You can't simply pick up your pre-fibromyalgia relationship. Nor should you want to continue the type of bond you developed when you were unhealthy.

Your being healthy will change the way other people relate to you. Don't assume family and friends will still chauffeur you, shop for you, or find time to listen to your everyday troubles now that you're healthy or close to it. It's risky to assume, expect, or demand too much.

Here's another warning: Don't be shocked if others don't welcome your healthy self with open arms and ample understanding. Some will persist in treating you as if you were still sick. Your spouse may need reminders not to continue to make decisions without "bothering" you. Your married children may have to be told repeatedly that visits with the grandchildren no longer set off an attack. You may have to phone old friends and talk just "happy talk"—and even then, they may still avoid you. That's life. Accept it, deal with it, and then move on. Having recovered from fibromyalgia, you know how silly it is to risk any part of your well-being worrying or getting angry about the past.

THURSDAY: START USING YOUR BODY AGAIN

Many of Dr. Selfridge's new patients admit that for years they've avoided exercise in order to avoid pain, because moving hurts. Unfortunately, becoming a couch potato can aggravate fibromyalgia. Dr. Selfridge remembers, "Back when medical research started showing that people with fibromyalgia should exercise, I realized I'd be in pain whether I sat or ran." She decided to try exercising more—running, cross-country skiing, and biking—and soon was competing in bike and triathlon events. She got so much pleasure from pushing her body to its limit that good neuropeptides flooded away her pain.

When Dr. Selfridge urged Betsy to get up, get out, and get around, Betsy took action. In addition to working nearly full time again, she now puts in twenty minutes a day on a treadmill and swims laps in her home pool. It sounds mighty rigorous, but Betsy feeds her incentive to keep going with a look in the mirror: "When I stick to this routine, I wear dresses that are two sizes smaller." Anna started walking four miles three days a week. She likes the solitude and fresh air and enjoys rubbing elbows with nature along her path, but she is also spurred on by the knowledge that inactivity allows pain-generating chemicals to initiate. The exercise gives her more than just physical conditioning; it also boosts her mentally.

We insist you check with your physician before beginning any exercise program. If you're pronounced fit, start today to exercise as long and vigorously as you can, in accordance with your doctor's guidelines. If you're already working out three times a week for at least thirty minutes each time, that's sufficient for now. But if you're under sixty, work up to one hour three times a week or half an hour five times a week.

If you have gone months without exercise, start with ten to fifteen minutes of walking. Being overweight is not an excuse. Get your heart pumping and your lungs breathing faster than normal. The increased oxygen and blood flow help to strengthen your muscles and, at the same time, provide nutrients for your brain and other organs. By the end of this week, work your way up to at least twenty minutes of continuous movement. Over a month, work up to at least thirty minutes at a stretch unless you need to accommodate a physical condition other than fibromyalgia. When in doubt, ask a physician for guidance, but be scrupulously honest when you describe your symptoms. Show your doctor this chapter, especially if you're over sixty, and explain that you're ready to start working your body again so that it will start working for you.

If you want exercise more vigorous than walking and your doctor okays it, go for it. If you can get to a health club or YMCA, check out circuit training or aerobics classes; they help tone muscle and condition your heart and lungs. If you jog, take care to protect your knees and hips by wearing good running shoes and running on soft ground. Or ride a bike (please wear a helmet!). Water aerobics is great for former couch potatoes: in soothing, cushioning water, an instructor leads you through a vigorous workout. Regularly scheduled water (or floor) aerobics programs provide great incentive for you to show up and work out. The esprit de corps you'll soon form with instructors and others in the group can be an effective motivator.

Try different exercise methods until you find what suits you. Don't be afraid to quit early when you need to or to make other accommodations to your changing health. Franklynn took part in a health club's hour-long water aerobics class. After forty-five minutes he would get chilled, so he'd hop out of the swimming pool and dash to a nearby hot whirlpool. From there he could still see the instructor, and he'd continue as best he could. Nobody complained.

To gauge how well you're retraining your body for health, let's set some goals for you. Start by taking your resting pulse rate (beats per minute) ten times today. (You don't have to count for a full minute if you have a clock or watch with an easy-to-read second hand. For six seconds count your pulse, then multiply by ten.) Always take your pulse after you've been sitting at least five minutes. Write the ten different readings on the accompanying chart, Goal-Setting to Get Your Heart and Lungs Working Again. Then take pulse readings during the middle of each exercise period for the next two months and keep a record of these.

What we want to accomplish by setting goals during your workouts is to get you back into good physical *and* mental condition within a reasonable time frame. So many people in the grip of fibromyalgia, for obvious reasons, don't exercise their bodies. Our bodies, brains, and minds are so interrelated that ignoring the physical workouts compromises your brains and minds. To achieve good results from your workouts, you should exercise not only your arms and legs, but your heart and lung muscles as well. By pushing yourself gradually to a point where your heart pumps up to 150 percent of your resting heart rate, you ensure that your heart and lungs are also benefiting from your exercise program.

If at any point during exercise you feel faint, numb, or dizzy, or if you experience pain, stop immediately. Sit or lie down and try to lower your head below heart level. Breathe deeply until you've recovered. Report your symptoms to your doctor right away and ask for guidance. This program is all about listening to your body's signals, so don't ignore warnings that you're overdoing it.

GOAL-SETTING TO GET YOUR HEART AND LUNGS WORKING AGAIN

	READING	RESTING PULSE RATE
	1	
	2	
	3	
	4	
	5	
	6	
	7	
	8	
	9	
	10	
Total of 10 numbers	A	
Divide A by 10 to get average resting pulse	B	
10% of B	C	
Month 1: Resting + 10% (C + B)	D	
Month 2: Resting + 20% (D + C)	E	
Month 3: Resting + 30% (E + C)	F	
Month 4: Resting + 40% (F + C)	G	
Month 5: Resting + 50% (G + C)	H	

Here's the most important reason for you to take your body off the couch and exercise it: When you exercise regularly, you double the attack on your fibromyalgia symptoms. You give your mind and body a strong message that you know the symptoms are temporary and reversible.

A WORD ABOUT PHYSICAL THERAPIES

Many fibromyalgia patients use various complementary treatments (physical therapy, massage, acupuncture, craniosacral manipulation, etc.) to manage their symptoms. Dr. Sarno found early in his practice that his patients didn't improve using the mind-body approach to their symptoms if they continued to use such physical treatment modalities. He discourages use of any physical treatments for TMS while his patients are using the mind-body method. We can understand why they might be counterproductive: While you're saying in your mind that emotions cause your symptoms, your actions in continuing these physical treatments suggest that you still believe, at least partially, that there's a reason to stay focused on your body.

Dr. Selfridge enjoys massage therapy. While she discontinued it for a while when she was applying Dr. Sarno's principles, she's recently resumed her weekly sessions. The difference is that when she goes now, it's with the goal of pampering her healthy mind-body rather than hoping the massage will give her temporary relief from pain. This change in purpose changes the outcome.

When God loves a creature, he wants the creature
to know the highest happiness and the deepest
misery. . . . He wants him to know all that being alive
can bring. That is his best gift. . . . There is no happiness save in understanding the whole.

—Thornton Wilder

14 WEEK FIVE: MAKE YOUR FREEDOM FROM FIBROMYALGIA LAST

Congratulations. You can soon put your painful
past behind you. You've come a long way toward
freedom from fibromyalgia, and you've done
the work on your own. A bright future beckons
ahead. Get on with your life.

If you're a quick healer and you've
found your symptoms disappearing as you've
worked your way up to here, it's time to make
plans to manage your health when you're
well. If you're close to getting well but not
sure you're at least 90 percent better, pay special attention to this week's exercises. Many
fibromyalgia sufferers never completely lose all
their symptoms, but the residue that remains is
insignificant compared to how it felt when
fibromyalgia ruled. If a symptom crops up, it's

often a reminder to deal with current emotion before it buries itself.

If your fibromyalgia is stubborn and won't let go, you may need substantially longer than five weeks to get the upper hand. Reread this book. Savor our encouragement. Work relentlessly to figure out what it is in your past, present, and daily life that's fighting to keep you in pain. In time you too are almost certain to regain your health.

You may want to seek a guide to help you. A psychotherapist trained in analysis (either Freudian or Jungian) can help you look for more conscious evidence of the unconscious processes that fed your fibromyalgia— but a behavioral psychotherapist is seldom as good a choice, and much of modern psychotherapy aimed at short-term intervention uses a behavioral approach. Behavior therapy examines and hopes to influence actions independently of the thoughts and emotions behind them, and by now you know enough about mind-body medicine to realize that separating actions from causative emotions is useless in getting rid of fibromyalgia symptoms.

Two attributes are most important in the guide you select: an understanding that you need to reflect deeply on the emotions governing your life, and the training to help you along. In our experience, therapists with these attributes are increasingly difficult to find. They're not cheap either—and managed health care is disinclined to pay for therapy that's for "personal growth" or "long-term" (more than a few sessions) despite its promise to eliminate costly doctor bills, procedures, and pills. We hope HMOs and insurance providers will catch up with modern mind-body theory some day.

You may have to "interview" the therapist on the phone before scheduling an appointment. You will want to ask about experience and skill with depth psychology and psychoanalysis. You may want to question the therapist's willingness to read Dr. Sarno's book, *The Mindbody Prescription*, and this book too. You can ask if the therapist has been trained in Freudian analysis or at one of the Jungian training institutes. If you understand this mind-body model (and you should be an expert by now), you may have to explain it to see how receptive the therapist is to your needs.

WHAT DO WE MEAN BY "CURED"?

There is no such thing as a 100 percent cure for fibromyalgia, just as there's not a 100 percent cure for our bones getting older, our teeth losing their luster, or our hair going gray. Dr. Selfridge feels 90 percent cured. Franklynn says he's at least that much better. Other patients pick similar numbers, almost all of them at or above 90 percent. They all feel, with few exceptions, that they've beaten back the pain so thoroughly, it no longer intrudes on life's activities.

What hangs around? Some of the lesser symptoms you had that are annoying but not incapacitating or terribly distracting. And the symptoms, when they occur, seem to go away as soon as you direct your thinking at your emotions. If you had restless legs, where your legs feel shot through with pins and needles and simply won't hold still, especially while trying to fall asleep, you may still have some of that. For some reason it doesn't go away as quickly as the knockout fibromyalgia pain does, but even when it doesn't go away entirely, it's generally much milder than before. It might simply show up a few times a month for no apparent reason. This is Franklynn's major aftereffect. His twitchy legs plague him if he lets himself nap close to bedtime, so he tries to keep from falling asleep while watching TV by sitting in a hard wooden rocker.

Another symptom often slow to disappear is sleep disturbance. It can take many months before you're consistently sleeping soundly. Try not to worry about it or expect changes too fast. The more pressure you put on yourself to get back to so-called normal sleep, the less likely you are to sleep easily and deeply. Instead, keep in mind that once you've licked the pain of fibromyalgia, you are very much a brand-new person. The new you might sleep less or more than the old you. Accept what the treatment gives you as being your new normal sleep pattern, and relax. A pattern takes time to establish itself.

Anna still hasn't returned to eight hours of sleep a night. She doesn't know if she ever will. But it's not a big deal any longer because she now gets five good hours, and that has become sufficient for her to carry on her normal life. She's turned the deficit into an advantage, one that gives her a couple of extra hours a day to enjoy her pain-free life.

Another common symptom that sometimes re-asserts itself is fatigue. Some tiredness revisits Dr. Self-ridge whenever she works in her garden. She expects and accepts it, saying, "That's only a few days a year—and I enjoy gardening so much." She's grateful she can garden again, something she couldn't enjoy at all for years.

When things get particularly stressful for Dr. Self-ridge, she gets acid reflux, another common fibromyal-gia symptom. But when it happens, she quickly talks back to the pain—"What's so important that you need my attention?"—and it goes away.

You too may have some annoying leftovers from your bout with fibromyalgia. Don't let them throw you or take you by surprise. Don't panic. You are still basi-cally in control. Meditate, journal; use self-talk, dreams, and exercise to stop your mind-body from manufac-turing any more of the biochemicals that cause fibro-myalgia.

Even pain may reassert itself from time to time, especially if you've been under a lot of stress. It's as if the fibromyalgia is testing you to see if you're still open to attack. If it happens, pull out your best counterattack—journal, meditation, self-talk—and chase it away.

Hold on to your goals and stick with the program. You can do it!

Fifty-three-year-old Helen, married and a grandmother, doesn't feel healed. There are still episodes when her fibromyalgia demon gets in the way. Like a spiteful enemy, fibromyalgia intrudes from time to time, mostly when she's got plans to do something special, such as go on vacation or celebrate somebody's birthday. Maybe that's why she still clings to her illness. She trained as a scientist and enjoys keeping up with the scientific journals. But perhaps because of her show-me nature, she keeps wondering, "If the treatment's that simple, why does anybody get fibromyalgia in the first place?"

If you're like Helen, we hope this book has helped answer that question for you. We prefer to phrase it positively: Since the treatment is so simple, why can't everybody get better? The path to freedom from fibromyalgia is a progression of simple sessions assembled into an overall plan.

We know the challenges you'll likely face as you work through this method, the doubters who'll protest, "If you get well practically overnight, you couldn't have been sick in the first place." One reason we asked you to read this book several times is to refresh its impact, so that you can continue to believe in and work your way toward health.

WORK YOU SHOULD ACCOMPLISH DURING WEEK FIVE

Our emphasis this week is on shifting your entire mindset from feeling clobbered by fibromyalgia to feeling nearly well again. For some people, it's a tough transition. After years of compensating for pain, fatigue, and general malaise, it can be a challenge to adapt your outlook to feeling no pain, more energy, and bright possibilities for the future.

○ Reread Chapter 13 for some tips on what you can do to behave like a well person.

○ Pick one more big aspect of life to simplify, and simplify it this week.

○ Plan to meditate on goals that can most help you make the transition to being well again. Think about relationships still in turmoil or still causing confusion. Don't forget to spend some time each day reflecting on emotions.

○ Redirect your journaling from illness to wellness. Pick at least one situation that shows your wellness. Describe it in detail.

○ Does it look like you need more time to heal? If so, use some meditation and journaling time to plan your extended treatment sessions. Guess how many more weeks you think it might take, and write that goal in your journal. If you need to prepare schedule sheets, do so now.

○ For the weekend session(s), unless you're extending for additional weeks, finalize your treatment details in your journal. Write about what you learned about yourself, what you learned about significant people in your life, which people became more significant and which became less. Examine your current or future job and your work at home. Plan how you will manage your new undertakings. This will minimize the chances of ever falling back into fibromyalgia again.

HOW TO SCHEDULE ASSIGNMENTS IF YOU TAKE LONGER

We set up our basic assignments to run for five weeks. Dr. Selfridge's experience shows it's about average for her patients. What's really important is how you feel. The point is not to put undue pressure on yourself. Don't demand miracles overnight. If at the end of five weeks you feel significantly better but not yet recovered from fibromyalgia, schedule several more weeks of practice in our methods. Eight weeks total is a fair goal for many people.

If you're going past our five-week schedule, for Week Six start with our schedule for Week Three, concentrating on what you now believe most needs the work. For Week Seven, revise the details in our schedule for Week Four. If you need more time, keep alternating and revising the schedules for Weeks Three and Four.

When you're feeling really well and are ready to wrap up your self-treatment, base your last week's assignments on our schedule for Week Five. It probably won't need much revision.

DON'T MAKE DRASTIC CHANGES YET

Early in this book we warned you away from making drastic changes in any part of your life while working through our assignments. We still don't want you to drastically change your meds, diet, or anything else of that magnitude. It's natural to want to dump every trace of the old life quickly and live only the new life, but that can result in a setback. Instead, gradually experiment with one change at a time. It's okay to proceed to cut back on tranquilizers, sleeping pills, braces, ointments, and the like if you believe you may no longer need them, as long as you have your doctor's approval. But be ready to restore any regimen whose loss seems to set you back—and remember that discontinuing medication abruptly can be harmful.

We strongly recommend that you go about it this way: Sit down with your journal and make a list of all the medications, herbs, nutritional supplements, diets, and special foods you're using now and want to modify. Show this list to your doctor and agree on what you can change. As you test each modification, make notes with dates. This way, if you suddenly find yourself feeling lousy again, you can quickly reconstruct a possible cause.

Dr. Selfridge has noticed that many people forget to take some of their medications when they have pain-free hours or days. This may be a clue that a particular medication can be reduced or eliminated. However, some medications commonly prescribed for fibromyalgia should not be dropped suddenly. Always consult a physician before tapering off or quitting. When Anna healed from fibromyalgia and tried cutting out her antidepressant, she found that she still suffers from clinical depression. She now expects to take Prozac or a comparable antidepressant the rest of her life, and accepts that her depression may never have been a part of her fibromyalgia, just coexistent with it.

It's risky even to make quick changes in your diet. People who've suffered with fibromyalgia for years have probably experimented with all kinds of diets. Franklynn dropped all artificial food additives when he was desperate to ease his pain. He still steers clear of them, believing that—even recovered—he is healthiest eating additive-free foods.

If you felt sad and tired with fibromyalgia, the feelings will disappear only if fibromyalgia caused them. If they're caused by a physical ailment, they won't go away.

People with TMS, including those with fibromyalgia, often report depression or anxiety symptoms worsening as their pain starts to go away. Dr. Sarno has found substitute symptoms occurring even after all the pain in an area is gone. If you experience greater depression or anxiety now that you're almost pain-free, try redoubling your efforts to focus on buried emotions. Don't be surprised if for a while you swing between pain and depression until your brain finally surrenders both symptoms.

REMAIN ALERT AND ASSERTIVE

For the next full year of your life, you'll need to make certain that you remain on top of fibromyalgia. Schedule all of the following simple tasks, and do them.

○ *Monitor your anger.* Once a month, make a journal entry of at least five pages on how you successfully identified and processed anger this month. Be specific. (If you don't remember any, great! Just make sure that you have been diligently looking.)

○ *Be wary of relationships.* Monthly, write in your journal about any relationships that still cause problems. Be as specific as possible in defining the problems and the emotions connected with them. Then write about relationships that got better during the past month. You needn't go into as much detail here.

○ *Simplify your life.* Monthly, reexamine in your journal everything you simplified during your recovery period. If you are slipping back into complications, draw up a plan for regaining control.

○ *Normalize your life.* After six months, take out Part D of the My Past, Present, and Fibromyalgia-Free Future worksheet (page 91). Fill in the "Follow-up After Fibromyalgia" column. Also, in your journal describe:

1. How you feel about the parts of your life that are obviously back to health

2. Why other aspects of your life are still not happy and stress-free
3. How you feel about the areas in which you're doing better than ever before
   In each case, notice any emotions that come up, and be sure to write about them.

○ *Keep this book* and your journals and charts where you can refer to them if you need some boosting as time goes by.

Life should be good again—not simply as good as it used to be, but better. You're a new person now. Despite being tired, pained, depressed, and confused, and despite the frustration of getting conflicting advice from people who knew less about fibromyalgia than you do now, you prevailed. You survived. You found the strength, character, and will to heal, and you came out on the other side more alive than ever.

Be well!

1. NIH web site on fibromyalgia. http://www.nih.gov/niams/news/niams-05.htm on 11/15/00.
2. MSNBC web site article, 8/26/99, by Linda Carol. http://www.msnbc.com/news/304040.asp.
3. Nom Hadler, *Spine*, October 15, 1996, 21, 20, 2397–99.
4. D. L. Goldenberg, *Archives of Internal Medicine*, April 26, 1999, 778.
5. Ibid., 779.
6. *Fibromyalgia Frontiers* [newsletter] 4, 4 (1996).
7. G. W. Waylonis et al., *American Journal of Physical Medicine Rehabilitation* 73, 6 (1994), 406–8.
8. *Fibromyalgia Frontiers* [newsletter] 4, 4 (1996).
9. Interview with J. Sarno: August 23, 1999.
10. M. Kennedy et al., *Arthritis and Rheumatism* 39, 4 (1996), 684.
11. J. M. Mountz et al., *American Journal of the Medical Sciences* 315, 6 (1998), 386.
12. S. Hunt et al., *Journal of Rheumatology* 25, 5 (1998), 1024.
13. Goldenberg, 782.
14. Ibid., 777–80.
15. Ibid.
16. R. M. Bennett, *Rheumatic Disease Clinics of North America* 19, 1 (1993), 51.
17. R. W. Simms, *American Journal of the Medical Sciences* 315, 6 (1998), 346–50.
18. Goldenberg, 780.
19. A. C. Steele et al., *Journal of the American Medical Association* 269 (1993), 1812–6.
20. H. Moldofsky, cited in S. M. Harding, *American Journal of the Medical Sciences* 315, 6 (1998), 371.

21. U. Hemmeter et al., "Schlafstorungen bei chronischen Schmerzen und generalisierter Tenomyopathie," *Schweizerische Medizinische Wochenschrift* 125, 49 (1995), 2391–7.

22. Waylonis et al.

23. C. Pert, *Molecules of Emotion* (New York: Touchstone, 1999), 67.

24. I. J. Russell, *American Journal of the Medical Sciences* 315 (1998), 377–82; repeated in M. J. Schwarz et al., *Neuroscience Letters* 259, 3 (1999), 196–98.

25. Pert, 133–134.

26. Pert, 139.

27. D. Chopra, *Quantum Healing* (New York: Bantam, 1990), 55.

28. Pert, 188.

29. Chopra, 38.

30. Pert, 71.

31. Ibid., 82.

32. Chopra, 38.

33. Pert, 182.

34. Ibid., 183.

35. Ibid., 183–84.

36. Chopra, 66.

37. L. J. Crofford, *American Journal of the Medical Sciences* 315, 6 (1998), 359.

38. Pert, 137.

39. Chopra, 66.

40. Ibid., 90.

41. Ibid., 188.

42. Chopra, 189.

43. J. Sarno, *The Mindbody Prescription* (New York: Warner Books, 1998), xvii.

44. Crofford.

45. Pert, 141.

46. Sarno, 26–27. Some editing performed on Sarno's original.

47. L. Erdrich, *Tales of Burning Love* (New York: HarperCollins, 1996).

48. S. Covey, *The Seven Habits of Highly Effective People* (New York: Simon & Schuster, 1990).

49. Based on http://www.nmha.org/infoctr/factsheets/44.cfm. Very similar to material on the American Psychological Association's web site: http://www.apa.org/pubinfo/anger.html.

50. Pert, 290.

There aren't yet many resources to use with the mind-body approach to healing fibromyalgia. We've listed here the ones we can find as we go to press. We've also offered references to books, web sites, or associations that can be helpful at various stages of your recovery. If you find others, drop us a line (FM, 3006 Gregory Street, Madison, WI 53711-1847) or e-mail us (FM@CPAComputerReport.com).

ANGER

http://www.mnha.org   web site of the National Mental Health Association, where you can find especially useful techniques and suggestions for coping well with anger.

ASSERTIVENESS

The Highly Sensitive Person: How to Thrive When the World Overwhelms You, by Elaine N. Aron (Broadway Books, 1997). This psychologist focuses on helping sensitive, shy, inward-looking people cope with a world that too often rewards the aggressive and insensitive. Fibromyalgia sufferers very much tend to fit Aron's description of "sensitive people."

The Highly Sensitive Person's Workbook, by Elaine N. Aron (Broadway Books, 1999). If you found the Aron book above to be rewarding, you might gain extra momentum on your path to healing from fibromyalgia by adding this matching workbook to your treatment.

DREAMS

Exploring the World of Lucid Dreaming, by Stephen LaBerge and
Howard Rheingold (Ballantine, 1990). There's more about
dreams in this lively book than you may want or need to
know. But LaBerge offers specific techniques in dreaming
and dream management that can be helpful if you want to
engage in dream analysis or dream journaling as you
progress toward freedom from fibromyalgia.

EXERCISE

The Aerobics Way, by Kenneth H. Cooper (Bantam, 1977).

MEDITATION

Deepak Chopra, M.D., *Boundless Energy* (Three Rivers Press, 1995).
A book aimed at chronic fatigue syndrome in particular, and
lack of energy in general. Chopra stresses noninvasive, mind-
oriented exercises, and meditation in particular. You may find
useful guidance here for intensifying your own meditation
experience.

SCIENTIFIC AND MEDICAL BACKGROUND

The Mindbody Prescription, by John E. Sarno, M.D. (Warner Books,
1998). This is the most recently published book for lay
readers by the pioneering physician, teacher, and researcher.
In it, Sarno demonstrates how mind-body techniques can
bring relief from TMS ailments such as certain back pains,
ulcers and arthritis, repetitive stress disorder (carpal tunnel
syndrome), colitis, migraine headaches, and many others.

Mind over Back Pain, by John E. Sarno, M.D. (William Morrow,
1984). An earlier Sarno book that emphasizes treatment of
back conditions using mind-body techniques.

Healing Back Pain, by John E. Sarno, M.D. (Warner Books, 1991).
A more recent Sarno book that emphasizes treatment of back
conditions using mind-body techniques.

Molecules of Emotion, by Candace Pert (Scribners, 1997). Pert is
a world-class biomedical researcher who writes as well as
she researches. It can set you straight about thoughts, sensations, emotions, pain, and other processes.

Quantum Healing: Exploring the Frontiers of Mind/Body Medicine, by Deepak Chopra, M.D. (Bantam Books, 1989). An early book by one of the first physicians to use and teach the power of healing the body by focusing the mind. You may have seen some of Chopra's inspirational seminars on public television stations.

WEB SITES AND INTERNET NEWSGROUPS

alt.med.fibromyalgia An extremely busy source of current events, gossip, and one-on-one support group messages. It's too crowded and clubby for our personal comfort, and members who post the most messages seem very hooked on symptoms and physical palliatives and procedures; they've more than once rejected attempts at healing using mind-body methods. If you log on only once a day, expect to download hundreds of new messages.

alt.med.fibromyalgia A place to meet fellow fibromyalgia sufferers and their families. Logging on once a day results in only a few dozen messages, as a rule.

http://www.mnha.org Web site of the National Mental Health Association, where you can especially find useful suggestions for coping with anger.

SUPPLIES

Required:

Journal (bound, not loose-leaf; wide-ruled if possible). (Chapter 8).

Pens needed to fill in some forms (with a cushioned barrel if you have sore fingers). You mostly need black or blue, but also red (Chapter 9).

Pencils needed to fill in some forms (Chapter 4).

Alarm clock needed to time meditation sessions when you're starting (Chapter 5).

Possibly needed:

Music source to mask background noise. It can be a radio, tape or CD player, or computer (Chapter 6).

I will forever be indebted to Dr. John Sarno. He has inspired me with his perseverance and his unusual (for a physician) ability and willingness to think outside the box. His friend and ally, Dr. Doug Hoffmann, introduced me to Dr. Sarno's work initially, when I expressed a desire to get rid of my fibromyalgia symptoms once and for all. I credit Dr. Sarno and Dr. Hoffmann with my "cure," and I thank them for giving me back my life. I also have to thank my children, Leah and Rachel, for picking up the slack at home, when I locked myself in my bedroom for hours working on each manuscript revision. They literally ran the household for me and they make me proud. My mother, Betty, read Dr. Sarno's books, even though she does not have chronic pain, and she rendered useful insights and supported me as only a mother can. My friends and soul mates, Phil and Gina, listened endlessly as I obsessed over my frustrations with the "reigning paradigm," and they never complained. They remain bright, shining stars in my new pain-free life and they keep me laughing.

We also offer special thanks to the Crown/Three Rivers publishing gurus who patiently and cleverly pruned and grafted this project into its present form, especially to executive editor Betsy Rapoport and her assistant, Stephanie Higgs, and to senior production editor Cindy Berman. And to our literary agent, Al Zuckerman, who found them for us at a time when it seemed like nobody wanted to publish a book on fibromyalgia.

—Nancy Selfridge, M.D.

Acetylcholine, 45
Acid reflux, 242
Acupuncture, 210, 211
ADP (adenosine diphosphate),
    30
Adrenal gland, 62
Adrenaline, 131
Age, fibromyalgia and, 4, 6
Allergy, 16
"All in head" attitude, 6, 9, 40,
    210
American College of
    Rheumatology, 28
Amino acids, 37
AMP (adenosine
    monophosphate), 30
Amygdala, 43
Angelou, Maya, 112
Anger, 58–59, 85–87, 103, 115,
    126–146 (see also Five-
    Week Healing Plan)
  communicating, 143–144
  fear of, 139
  finding specific, 133–137
  journaling and, 148–150,
    167–169, 172
  List, 135–137, 211–212, 214,
    218, 221
  management of, 137–146

meditation on, 146
  One-Minute Anger Manager,
    140–141
  reaching for, 131–133
Antibodies, 36
Antidepressant drugs, 12, 37,
    210, 247
Antigens, 36
Arginine, 7
Aron, Elaine, 56
Assignment Scheduler, 153, 158
  first week, 189, 194–195
  second week, 196–197
  third week, 198–199
  fourth week, 200–201
  fifth week, 202–203
Associations, chain of, 145
ATP (adenosine triphosphate),
    30
Autonomic function center, 9,
    42, 43

Back pain, 22
Balance problems, 16
Baruch, Bernard, 204
Behavior therapy, 239
Bennett, Robert M., 31, 68
Bone marrow, 48
Brainstem, 42

Breathing, 120–121
Bruxism (grinding teeth), 16

Calcium, 37
Carlin, George, 24, 101
CCK, 51
Central nervous system, 36,
        40–41
    chemical messenger system,
        44–48
    classic nervous system, 42–44
    endocrine system, 47, 50–51
    immune system, 47, 48–50
Cerebral cortex, 43
Chemical messenger system,
        44–48
Chicken pox, 32
Childhood abuse, 15, 57, 59
Chopra, Deepak, 52–54, 174
Chronic fatigue syndrome, 11,
        14–15, 16
Churchill, Sir Winston, 208
Classic nervous system, 42–44
Cleaning house, 104
Clergy, 81
Coccyx pain, 16
Cold, sensitivity to, 35, 61
Cold sores, 16, 32
Concentration problems, 16
Constipation, 16
Cooking, 104, 107
Covey, Stephen, 144
Crofford, Leslie J., 62–63

Degenerative joint disease
        (DJD), 10
Depression, 11, 12, 16, 247
Diagnosis of fibromyalgia, 7–8,
        10–11
Diarrhea, 16
Directed meditation (see
        Meditation)
Disability insurance, 28, 72
Dopamine, 45
Dreams, 174–183, 218

    remembering, 176–178
    seeding, 180–183
    writing down, 177–179
Dynorphin A, 38

Echinacea, 7
Emotions, 49–50, 55, 58–60,
        64, 84 (see also Anger)
Endocrine system, 41, 47,
        50–51
Endorphins, 37, 38, 46, 51
Enkephalins, 38, 46
Epiphany, moment of, 224–225
Epstein-Barr virus (EBV), 31–32
Erdrich, Louise, 139
Estrogen, 41
Euler, Ulf von, 38
Euthanasia, 5
Exercise program, 232–237
Exploring the World of Lucid Dreaming
        (LaBerge and
        Rheingold), 178

Fascitis, 10
Feet, burning, 16
Fibro fog, 4–5, 12–14
Fibromyalgia
    age and, 4, 6
    "all in head" attitude toward,
        6, 9, 40, 210
    childhood abuse and, 15, 57,
        59
    conditions aggravating, 19–20
    diagnosis of, 7–8, 10–11
    dreams and (see Dreams)
    exercise program and,
        232–237
    fibro fog, 4–5, 12–14
    fibro-spot pain, 84–87, 140
    financial cost of, 7
    gender and, 4, 20, 62
    genetic susceptibility to, 33
    immune system and, 36, 41,
        47, 48–50
    incidence of, 4, 6–7

Fibromyalgia (cont'd)
  journaling and (see
    Journaling)
  Lyme disease and, 32, 33
  medications for, 88–89,
    246–247
  meditation and (see
    Meditation)
  metabolism and, 30–31
  muscles and, 29–31
  myths concerning, 24–38
  overlapping symptoms,
    10–12
  personal relationships and,
    72–74, 76–77, 79–82,
    110, 153, 216, 231–232
  positive attitude and, 67–71
  psychotherapy and, 57, 71,
    110, 239–240
  race and, 4
  self-talk and, 147, 162–164,
    166, 229
  simplifying life and, 80–81,
    101–111, 204–207,
    217, 219–220
  sleep disturbances and, 26,
    34–35, 210, 241–242
  stress and, 61–64, 70
  symptoms of, 4–5, 11–12,
    16–18
  treatment for (see Treatment
    plan)
  triggers, 58–61, 63, 70,
    128–130
  visualization and (see
    Visualization)
Fibro-spot pain, 84–87, 140
Financial cost of fibromyalgia, 7
Five-Week Healing Plan,
  187–249
  Week One, 187–195
  Week Two, 204–207
  Week Three, 208–222
  Week Four, 223–237
  Week Five, 238–249

Fluid retention, 16
Food additives, 247
Freedom from Fibromyalgia
  Assignment Scheduler
  (see Assignment
  Scheduler)
Freudian analysis, 239, 240
Frustration Index, 170

Gallbladder, 50, 51
Gastroesophageal reflux disease
  (GERD), 10
Gender, fibromyalgia and, 4, 20,
  62
Genetic susceptibility to
  fibromyalgia, 33
Goal-Setting to Get Your Heart
  and Lungs Working
  Again, 235, 236
Goethe, Johann Wolfgang von,
  174
Goldenberg, Don L., 28
Gonads, 50
Green, Elmer, 52
Grocery shopping, 104
Growth hormone, 51
Guilt, about anger, 131, 132

Hadler, Nortin M., 210
Hamilton, Sean F., 40
Headaches, 62, 210
Healing tools (see Dreams;
  Journaling; Meditation;
  Self-talk; Visualization)
Heat, sensitivity to, 16, 61
Herpes viruses, 32
Highly Sensitive Person, The (Aron),
  56
Hindbrain, 42
Hippocampus, 43
Historical Record of My Key
  Milestones, 83,
  158–160, 190
Holmes, Thomas, 128
Homework, 75

Hormones, 50, 51
Household chores, 107
HPA/HPG, 62
5HTP, 38
Hypothalamus, 62

"I" message, 143
Immune system, 36, 41, 47,
        48–50
Injuries, 35
Insulin, 41, 50
Ionesco, Eugène, 3
Iron, 37
Irritable bowel syndrome (IBS),
        10, 11, 61

Journaling, 143, 147–161 (see
        also Five-Week Healing
        Plan)
    anger, 148–150, 167–169,
        172
    changing entries, 156
    creating journal, 150–152
    dreams, 177–179, 182
    Historical Record of My Key
        Milestones, 158–160
    methods, 152–156
    My Fibromyalgia Time Line,
        158, 160–161
    revisionist, 169–173, 220,
        221
    revisiting journal, 167–169
    sample entry, 157
    topics, 154
Jungian analysis, 239, 240

Kennedy, Maura, 26
Kerkenham, Miles, 44
Kevorkian, Jack, 5
Kidneys, 48, 50

LaBerge, Stephen, 178
Lamaze childbirth method, 51
L-dopa, 37
Leeman, Susan, 38

Lidocaine, 5
Light, sensitivity to, 35
Limbic system, 22, 42–43, 64
Litigation, 72
Liver, 47, 48, 50
Locking diaries, 150
Loose-leaf binders, 151
Lupus (systemic lupus
        erythematosus, SLE),
        10–11
Lyme disease, 32, 33
Lymph nodes, 48
Lymphocytes (white blood
        cells), 36, 48, 49

Mantra, 121
Massage therapy, 237
Medications, 88–89, 246–247
Meditation, 14, 51, 112–125,
        143 (see also Five-Week
        Healing Plan)
    on anger, 146
    atmosphere for, 115–116
    breathing and, 120–121
    focus on focusing, 121–124
    relaxation and, 117–119
    time of sessions, 113, 115
Memory problems, 16
Metabolism, 30–31
Methadone, 5
Migraine, 11, 210
Mind-body connection, 40,
        52–54, 210–211
Mindbody Prescription, The (Sarno), 8,
        56, 128, 240
Mitochondria, 30
Mitral valve prolapse, 16
Moldofsky, Harvey, 13, 34
Molecules of Emotion (Pert), 174
Monocytes (white blood cells),
        49, 50
Mononucleosis, 32
Montagu, Ashley, 187
Motivational tapes, 113
Mountz, James M., 26–27

Muscle fatigue, 16
Muscles, 29–31
Music, for meditation, 116
My Fibromyalgia Time Line,
      158, 160–161, 190–191
Myofascial pain syndrome,
      10–12
Myofibril separation, 29
My Past, My Present, My
      Fibromyalgia-Free
      Future, 90–100, 153,
      190, 215, 216, 218,
      227–228, 248
Myths concerning fibromyalgia,
      24–38

National Institute of Arthritis
      and Musculoskeletal and
      Skin Diseases (NIAMS),
      4
National Institutes of Health, 28
Neck problems, 16
Neuropeptides
      (neurotransmitters), 9,
      21, 37, 41–42, 44–49,
      51, 52
Nietzsche, Friedrich, 126
Nitrous oxide, 37
No, use of, 106, 107
Noise, sensitivity to, 35, 61
Noradrenaline, 131
Norepinephrine, 45
Numbness, 11, 16, 17, 35, 241

One-Minute Anger Manager,
      140–141
Osteoarthritis, 10
Oxygen, in muscles, 31

Pain signals, 36–38
Palpitations, 16
Pancreas, 50
Paresthesia (pins and needles),
      11, 17, 35, 241
PCr (phosphocreatine), 31

Pelvic pain, 17, 35
Perfectionists and goodists,
      86–87, 104, 133, 151
Personal relationships, 72–74,
      76–77, 79–82, 110,
      231–232
Pert, Candace, 41, 44, 49–50,
      64, 174–176
Pins and needles, 11, 17, 35,
      241
Pituitary gland, 48, 50, 62
Positive attitude, 67–71, 112
Premenstrual syndrome (PMS),
      11, 17, 62
Priorities, setting, 106–107
Prolactin, 48
Prostaglandins, 37
Prozac, 247
Psychoneuroimmunology, 53
Psychotherapy, 57, 71, 110,
      239–240

Rage, 55, 58–59, 137 (see also
      Anger)
Rahe, Richard, 128
Relationship Planner, 73, 74,
      76–77, 153, 190, 191,
      216
Relaxation, 117–119
Repetitive-motion disorders, 35
Reproductive organs, 48, 62
Reptilian brain, 42
Resting pulse rate, 235, 236
Restless legs, 17, 26, 35, 241
Revisionist journaling, 169–173,
      220, 221
Rheingold, Howard, 178
Rheumatoid arthritis, 11, 12

St. John's wort, 38
Sarno, John E., 8, 22, 23, 26,
      28, 54–58, 72, 78, 86,
      109, 128, 237, 240, 247
Sarnoff, Stanley J., 209
Schizophrenia, 45

Sciatica, 17, 35
Seeding dreams, 180–183
Selenium, 37
Self-hypnosis, 112
Self-talk, 147, 162–164, 166,
    229
Serotonin, 37–38, 41
Sexual abuse, 57
Sexual dysfunction, 17, 35
Sicca symptoms (dry eyes, dry
    mouth), 11
Simplifications, 80–81,
    101–111, 204–207,
    217, 219–220
Sinus problems, 17
Sleep apnea, 34
Sleep disturbances, 17, 26,
    34–35, 210, 241–242
Spinal abnormalities, 210
Spinal blocks, 5
Spine (journal), 210
Spleen, 47, 48, 51
Status diagnosis, 8
Stomach ulcers, 17
Stress, 61–64, 70
    life events and, 128–130
Substance P, 38, 210
Support networks, 81
Swollen glands, 17
Symptoms of fibromyalgia, 4–5,
    11–12, 16–18
Synaptic cleft, 44

Tachycardia, 17, 35
Tales of Burning Love (Erdrich), 139
Temper tantrums, 132
Temporomandibular joint (TMJ)
    pain, 10, 17
Tendonitis, 10
Tension myositis syndrome
    (TMS), 22, 55–56, 247
Thyroid, 50
Time-out, 143
Tinnitus (ringing in ear), 17
Transferon, 50–51

Treatment plan, 187–249
    Goal-Setting to Get Your Heart
        and Lungs Working
        Again, 235, 236
    Historical Record of My Key
        Milestones, 83,
        158–160, 190
    My Past, My Present, My
        Fibromyalgia-Free
        Future, 90–100, 153,
        190, 215, 216, 218,
        227–228, 248
    Relationship Planner, 73, 74,
        76–77, 153, 190, 191,
        216
    time and space for, 75, 78,
        79–82
    Week One, 187–195
    Week Two, 204–207
    Week Three, 208–222
    Week Four, 223–237
    Week Five, 238–249
Triggers of fibromyalgia, 58–61,
    63, 70, 128–130
Tryptophan, 36

Urinary urgency, 11

Vertigo, 17
Visualization, 14, 82–83, 112,
    147, 164–166, 229
    of anger, 139
    breathing, 120
Volunteering activities, 105, 106

Welty, Eudora, 223
Wheelchairs, 105
White blood cells, 36, 48–50
Wilder, Thornton, 238
WordPad, 152
World Health Organization, 28

Xiao-Ming Tian, 19

Yoga, 51

NANCY SELFRIDGE, M.D., practices family medicine with the University of Wisconsin Health–Physicians Medical Group in Madison, specializing in treating fibromyalgia, and operates the Fibromyalgia Support Group.

FRANKLYNN PETERSON has written more than twenty self-help books.